1 Out of 10 Doctors Recommends

H. Eric Bender, MD,
Murdoc Khaleghi, MD,
and Bobby Singh, MD

1 Out of 10 Doctors Recommends

*Drinking Urine,
Eating Worms,
and Other Weird
Cures, Cases, and
Research from the
Annals of Medicine*

ST. MARTIN'S GRIFFIN
NEW YORK

www.stmartins.com

Designed by Jonathan Bennett

Library of Congress Cataloging-in-Publication Data

Names: Bender, H. Eric. | Khaleghi, Murdoc. | Singh, Bobby (Psychiatrist)
Title: 1 out of 10 doctors recommends : drinking urine, eating worms, and
  other weird cures, cases, and research from the annals of medicine / H.
  Eric Bender, MD, Murdoc Khaleghi, MD, and Bobby Singh, MD
Other titles: One out of ten doctors recommend
Description: First edition. | New York : St. Martin's Griffin, [2016] |
  Includes bibliographical references.
Identifiers: LCCN 2016003972| ISBN 9781250070579 (trade pbk.) |
  ISBN 9781250073136 (e-book)
Subjects: LCSH: Medical misconceptions. | Medicine—Humor.
Classification: LCC R729.9 .B46 2016 | DDC 610—dc23
LC record available at http://lccn.loc.gov/2016003972

Our books may be purchased in bulk for promotional, educational, or business use. Please contact your local bookseller or the Macmillan Corporate and Premium Sales Department at 1-800-221-7945, extension 5442, or by e-mail at MacmillanSpecialMarkets@macmillan.com.

First Edition: August 2016

10 9 8 7 6 5 4 3 2 1

To my parents, whose infinite love shines around me like a million blazing suns.

BOBBY

This book is dedicated to Laura, who somehow puts up with me. I also dedicate this to Andy, Alyssa, and PJ—I am lucky their mother did such a good job raising them. The three of you are the ultimate hat trick!

MURDOC

This book is dedicated to you, Mom. I wish you were here to see it.

ERIC

Contents

CONTENTS

CONTENTS

CONTENTS

Acknowledgments

Looking back, we recognize that the existence of this book is about as unlikely as us performing or undergoing most of the practices in this book. Which is why we would first like to thank our publisher, who by now should have known better than to take a chance on us again. Thank you, Daniela Rapp!

And when this book was rejected by multiple agents, we were fortunate to find an agent whose tastes were more in line with ours, even if that was unfortunate for our new agent. Thank you, Alison Fargis!

When we realized we weren't nearly as humorous as the topics in this book, we found a partner who shares our love of both humor and health. Thank you, Courtney Pong!

And when we needed some guidance on illustrations and those eye-catching pics, we could rely on the talented eyes of Nicole DiMella. Thank you, Nicole!

When we doubted whether people would be interested in these topics, our spouses pretended to be just interested enough to keep us going. Thank you, Sarah, Laura, and Sujatha! A huge thank-you also to the children in our lives (Maya, Kavi, Imogen, Andy, Alyssa, and PJ) for letting us sleep every other night undisturbed so we would stay sane long enough to finish this book.

Finally, thank you to our colleagues David Kim, MD, and Amit Raheja, MD, and to all our educators and mentors, some of whom inspired our creativity and humanity, and others who tried hard to beat it out of us, thereby making us work even harder to preserve it.

Introduction

It has often been said that nine out of ten doctors recommend this practice or that treatment. So, as practicing physicians, we were compelled to ask, "What the heck does that one other doctor recommend?"

1 Out of 10 Doctors Recommends finally solves that mystery.

This book draws from our medical education and clinical experiences. In fact, the idea for this book was born when one of the authors was a medical student on an internal medicine rotation. He sat at the computer scrolling through the medications listed in the electronic medical record system and happened upon "leeches." Not only did this surprise him, but the fact that research had been performed as to where on a patient leeches should be placed, including on the patient's *entire body*, seemed simply unbelievable.

Spurred on by this remarkable discovery, we have taken an engaging and humorous look at some of the strangest and most unusual medical practices, research, and case studies across time and cultures, including:

- *Performing fecal transplants to treat certain infections.*
- *Slapping body parts to get the same results as plastic surgery.*
- *Research demonstrating that skydiving might actually be dangerous.*
- *Applying maggots to heal wounds.*

- *Espousal of the safety and utility of heavy metals such as lead and mercury.*
- *Poking microscopic holes in your face to make you look younger.*

A further impetus for this book came from our realization that although the history of medicine is replete with research, recommendations, and remedies that might be considered unusual or just plain "crazy" by most people, there are equally as many contemporary outlandish practices. And what is perhaps most unbelievable: Many of these practices, research ideas, and treatments are grounded in valid science and/or actually seem to work. Others, however, have proven to be examples of medical quackery, and even dangerously wrong in certain cases.

As three physicians specializing in fields that include child, adolescent, adult, and geriatric mental health, as well as emergency medicine, we bear witness on a daily basis to the age-old irony of clinical care: Patients complain that doctors never listen, and doctors complain that patients never follow doctors' recommendations. *1 Out of 10 Doctors Recommends* suggests potential reasons why some patients might choose to disregard the counsel of their so-called highly educated and extensively trained physicians.

But from our diverse practices and numerous patients, we have learned that regardless of diagnosis or prognosis, humor is often the best medicine. Readers will certainly find the humor here. The best medicine part . . . we'll let you be the judge.

1

The Creepiest of All Treatments

Ever had a cut that just does not seem to get better? Ever wonder what you might have to do if it doesn't heal? Stop wondering, as you may then decide it's not worth fixing.

Before getting to the dirty truth, it's worth knowing how to avoid getting into this sort of situation. Our bodies naturally have an amazing ability to heal themselves, an ability we have evolved—or "intelligently designed," some might say—over millions of years. We tend to heal fairly quickly, making us just slightly slower versions of Wolverine.

We are not all so fortunate, though. Blood flow is essential to healing, as it carries various nutrients to the injured tissue. Anything that interferes with blood flow, such as vascular disease or diabetes, can impair our ability to heal. The simplest wounds can cause tissue to die and become infected, prompting more tissue death and infection. If only there were some way to get rid of dead tissue, or more specifically, something that could *eat* dead tissue—other than zombies.

Enter the maggots. Since the 1930s, doctors have observed that maggots can help remove infected and dead tissue from wounds. Soon after, they came up with something even better to kill bacteria: antibiotics. So unfortunately, the tiny worms fell out of favor. We became hooked on the antibiotics, as we do on many drugs, and started using them excessively. As a result, the last two decades have seen the emergence of antibiotic-resistant "superbugs." As we have learned from SyFy-channel movies, the best way to fight superbugs is with other bugs. Reenter the maggots.

Now maggot therapy is used at more than eight hundred health care institutions, and maggots can be readily prescribed as a regulated medical device. Apparently, even maggots can't escape bureaucracy. We do not know what the charge is for maggot therapy, but we assume there is an impressive markup, making one man's trash another man's treasure. Maggots are especially helpful in preventing infections from getting past knees and elbows, as they congregate well in those areas. Perhaps maggots like to hang out in knees and elbows so they can ask each other, "What's a nice maggot like you doing in a joint like this?"

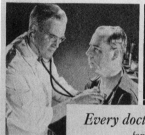
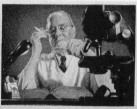
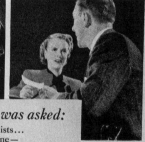

Every doctor in private practice was asked:
—family physicians, surgeons, specialists...
doctors in every branch of medicine—
"What cigarette do you smoke?"

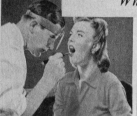
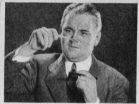
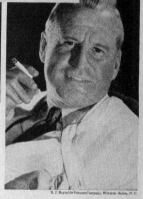

According to a recent Nationwide survey:

More Doctors
Smoke Camels

than any other cigarette!

R. J. Reynolds Tobacco Company, Winston-Salem, N. C.

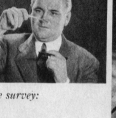

THE
"T-ZONE" TEST
WILL
TELL YOU

The "T-Zone"—T for taste and T for throat—is your own laboratory, your proving ground, for any cigarette. For only your taste and your throat can decide which cigarette tastes best to you...and how it affects your throat. On the basis of the experience of many, many millions of smokers, we believe Camels will suit your "T-Zone" to a "T."

Not a guess, not just a trend...but an actual fact based on the statements of doctors themselves to 3 nationally known independent research organizations.

Yes, your doctor was asked...along with thousands and thousands of other doctors from Maine to California. And they've named their choice—the brand that more doctors named as their smoke is *Camel!* Three nationally known independent research organizations found this to be a fact.

Nothing unusual about it. Doctors smoke for pleasure just like the rest of us. They appreciate, just as you, a mildness that's cool and easy on the throat. They too enjoy the full, rich flavor of expertly blended costlier tobaccos. And they named Camels...more of them named Camels than any other brand. Next time you buy cigarettes, try Camels.

1946 Advertisement for Camel Cigarettes. More Doctors Smoke Camels. Obtained from The Granger Collection, New York.

2

More Doctors Smoke Camels . . . Well, What Else Would You Do to a Camel?

As cigarette smoking rose in popularity in the 1930s and 1940s, an equally large concern in the medical community loomed about the negative effects of smoking. In order to combat the growing worry among the public, cigarette companies' advertising agencies began to picture physicians in ads for their products, reminding us of why we love *Mad Men*. In 1946, one of the most iconic advertisements pictured a man in a white coat holding a cigarette and smiling. The words printed alongside the picture read, "According to a recent Nationwide survey: More Doctors Smoke Camels than any other cigarette!" This guy was presumably a doctor, although when did you last see your doctor smile?

It turns out that the marketing group for the cigarette company conducted this "nationwide survey" at medical conferences and in physicians' offices right after providing the doctors with complimentary cartons of Camels. The "researchers" then asked the doctors which brand of cigarettes they preferred or had in their pockets. And you thought pharmaceutical reps were bad!

Perhaps so as not to just focus on the public's concern about health issues, some cigarette companies also tried to allay anxiety over physical appearance. A 1929 ad for Lucky Strike cigarettes showed a woman puckering her face, bearing the world's first official Duck Face, below the words "To keep a slender figure no one can deny . . . Reach for a Lucky instead of a sweet." A 1949 ad for Viceroy Filtered Cigarettes pictured a dentist who held a dental mirror and exclaimed, "As your Dentist I would recommend Viceroys." Luckily most people don't listen to their dentists anyway.

If we look beyond vintage advertising, even in our clinical experience we have run across patients whose doctors talked to them about cigarettes, but not in the way you'd hope. One of our colleagues saw a man who had pica as a child. Pica is the persistent eating of substances that are nonnutritive, such as sand, clay, gravel, glass, paper, or other materials. In order to get the patient to stop his pica, the patient's pediatrician told him to start smoking cigarettes. So he did. At age five. Because the taste of a cigarette is better post-afternoon story time and naps.

3

Stuck on You

If you've ever watched *Stand By Me*, you probably remember the horrific scene after the four boys wade through the swamp when Gordie, played by Wil Wheaton, reaches into his tighty-whities and pulls out a leech. It's hard to imagine, but some medical doctors actually order leeches to be applied to various parts of the body—though typically not the part Gordie's leech glommed on to.

Leeches use suckers on their bodies to attach to their hosts and consume the host's blood. For this reason, in medieval times, leeches were used in the process of bloodletting. Bloodletting was performed to balance the four humors, or bodily fluids, believed to affect one's health and disposition. We can't imagine that having leeches suck your blood would balance anything. In modern times, however, leeches have been used to prevent clots, because they naturally produce a blood thinner. This innate blood thinner is one reason that leeches themselves don't die right away after they gulp and guzzle a bunch of blood.

Dr. David Kim, a plastic-surgeon colleague of ours, told us of the involvement of leeches in his practice—and he wasn't talking about insurance companies. He explained that leeches can be used to decrease venous congestion in patients who have had tissue transfers. Venous congestion is the number one cause of failure immediately following such procedures, because congested blood can stagnate, leading to decreased fresh blood flow into the tissue. Leeches provide new outlets for congested blood, allowing arteries to deliver nutrient-rich blood. Ta-da! The tissue is saved.

Dr. Kim even described his method of applying the cute little guys. He cuts a hole in the bottom of a coffee cup and then directs the leeches out of the hole toward their destination. "Those guys are really fast!" he added. "With this method, you avoid having to chase leeches all around a patient's room." While it's hard to imagine this happening, we like to think that "Yakety Sax" (think Benny Hill) plays when it does.

Just be glad you're not a medical student on Dr. Kim's service—and double-check to be sure you picked up the right coffee cup.

4

Want Fries with That?

Medical-school lore often includes the tale of a woman who went to see her family practitioner exclaiming that she had "flowers growing down there." When the doctor checked, sure enough, she had leaves between her legs. Upon further examination, the "flowers" were found to be sprouting from a source a few inches inside of her: a potato. The woman, whom you might expect to be shocked, actually remembered having the potato placed in her vagina after she had given birth to stop the bleeding.

While this sounds absolutely vile, there might be some basis for the use of spuds to stop bleeding. Per some research, microporous polysaccharide hemispheres (MPH), or potato starch, may dehydrate blood and accelerate clotting. In one study, MPH decreased the time that it took for bleeding to stop in rats whose femoral arteries were pierced. In fact, there is a hemostatic product called Bleed-X, made in part from potato starch, that helps to stop bleeding in certain types of bleeding disorders in humans. There have been reports of potato-based powders that stop bleeding in small cuts on the forearm as well. This spud's for you.

Rat arteries and small cuts are one thing, but postnatal potato insertion is clearly another. So what happened to the woman with a spud in her birth canal? Well, the potato was removed, and typical vaginal flora was able to grow in place of what had clearly been an atypical vaginal floral arrangement.

5

Unwrinkling a Wizard's Sleeve?

Botox. It's been all the rage in Hollywood for years. Thanks to this neurotoxin produced by the bacterium *Clostridium botulinum*, everyone from Heidi Montag to your local newscaster can prohibit their true emotions from showing when pondering the demise of their careers.

Botulinum toxin, otherwise known as Botox, is a protein that can interfere with signals sent through the nervous system. As a result, the muscles that are downstream from those inhibited nerve impulses become as dysfunctional as Sarah Palin talking about . . . anything. When too much of the toxin is present, an illness called botulism can occur. The most common type of botulism occurs in children under age one: floppy-baby syndrome, and it can be fatal. This syndrome occurs when these children ingest something, such as honey or microscopic dust particles, that contains spores of the *Clostridium botulinum* bacterium. The young child's large intestine is ripe for germination of the spores and production of the toxin, leading to floppy-baby syndrome.

Injection of controlled amounts of the toxin can have a cosmetic purpose. When facial muscles are paralyzed, fewer wrinkles are visible, and one would also expect fewer wrinkles in the future. However, when excessive "controlled" amounts of Botox are used, you can end up looking like that star of *Real Housewives*. Yes, it is the one you are thinking of, as it doesn't really matter whom you are thinking of.

In reality, Botox has tremendous therapeutic use that is often overshadowed by its reputation among the stars. Botox can frequently relieve conditions such as blepharospasm (excessive blinking), hemifacial spasm (spasm of half the face), and torticollis (head and neck spasms). Botox is also used to treat vaginismus, which is a physical or psychological condition that results in uncontrollable vaginal muscle spasms upon vaginal penetration. In fact, one doctor treats this condition often enough to want to stake his claim on the practice with a website, vaginismusMD.com. Maybe this is the modern-day equivalent of having the "Assman" license plate in that *Seinfeld* episode.

You would think that having your genitals injected with a toxin would cause increased psychological and physical trauma, but the relief from this treatment has been reported to be quite effective and to last up to ten months in some cases. There is no report on whether repeated treatments lead to floppy-vagina syndrome.

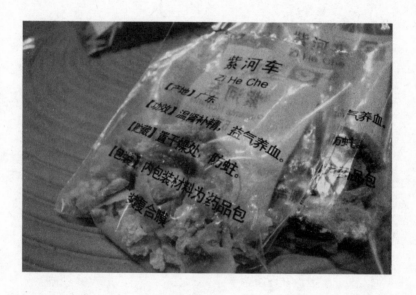

Human Placenta, Dried and Packaged.
From Wikimedia Commons.

6

Placenta: It's Not Just for Breakfast Anymore

Next to the baby that grows inside a pregnant woman's uterus is the placenta, an organ with a vast network of blood vessels that supplies the fetus with nutrients necessary for it to develop. At birth, the newborn seems to get all the attention, and most people forget about the placenta, in much the same way as we all forgot that *Friends* had a *Joey* spin-off. In fact, the baby's once indispensable womb-mate is frequently called the "afterbirth" and gets relegated to a lowly bucket—but not always.

Some mothers, and some unsuspecting fathers who get dragged into this, are consuming some of the placenta after birth. According to the United Kingdom's Independent Placenta Encapsulation Network (IPEN)—yes, that exists—the practice of eating placenta, also called placentophagy, has been a part of traditional Chinese medicine for centuries. Modern spins on this age-old practice are reflected in creative cuisine: placental pills, ice cubes, soups, and even pizza topping.

Why eat this seemingly unappetizing organ? Some believe that the placenta is rich in iron and other nutrients that can benefit the adult as well as the baby. Others claim that placental ingestion decreases postpartum depression, improves energy, and enhances breast-milk production. For a fee, IPEN will take a chunk of the placenta and make capsules or a smoothie, if you prefer. Watch out, Jamba Juice!

Despite the anecdotal reports of the effects of placental ingestion, formal studies do not show any significant benefits. On the other hand, we haven't seen studies showing harmful effects, either. So don't let us get in the way. Actually, does anyone else envision the next great Quickfire challenge on *Top Chef*?

7

Does This Jersey Make Me Look Fat?

Fans of the National Football League (NFL) give their hearts, their souls, and extremely large sums of money to their teams. According to a study by professor of marketing Pierre Chandon, NFL fans also give up their girlish figures. In the (incredibly lengthy-titled) study "From Fan to Fat? Vicarious Losing Increases Unhealthy Eating, but Self-Affirmation Is an Effective Remedy," Chandon reveals that the day after their team loses, particularly when it loses by a narrow margin, football fans eat more and eat up to 28 percent more saturated fats, like butters and meats, than they typically would. On the flip side, fans eat up to 16 percent fewer fatty foods after a victory.

Some fans have recognized a change in their eating habits and waistlines throughout the season and admit to chomping down on fatty foods—everything from pizza to Hot Pockets. So why do they do it? And why are people still eating Hot Pockets?

Researchers suggest that fans might use eating as a coping mechanism when their identities are threatened after a loss. Well, it's no surprise that NFL fans do identify with their teams; just look at the Black Hole in Oakland. We have no idea what—or who—that crew eats after a loss.

It's also true that this could be comfort eating, which people frequently do—you know who you are. Recall *The Golden Girls* and their cheesecake habit? But even more realistically, c'mon, would you rather eat a cinnamon roll or a salad? The answer is pretty much going to be the same any day of the week, no?

Not necessarily, when it comes to your football team. Per Chandon, after your team wins, you feel strong enough about yourself to "delay gratification and resist temptation." This then explains why fans in Cleveland and Buffalo aren't exactly known as the sultans of svelte.

8

A Sting to Treat a Sting

When you hear the term "venom," our guess is you typically think poison rather than cure (although the second-most-common association seems to be "Ann Coulter," based on an informal survey we did). While many products have been promoted as cure-alls, not many are nearly as promoted, or as scary, as bee venom. In fact, the medical use of honeybee products is so promoted that it has its own term—"apitherapy"—to make it sound less unpleasant. There is even an American Apitherapy Society and so of course a *Journal of the American Apitherapy Society*. We question whether they might be a little biased for the bee venom in the research they publish.

Honeybee-venom therapy has been promoted as a treatment for viruses, autoimmune diseases, cancer, multiple sclerosis, arthritis, scars, and nearly everything else—all but the treatment of allergic reaction to bee stings and a bad case of lovin' you.

Unlike many panaceas, honeybee venom actually does have some evidence for effectiveness in very specific settings. For example, a toxin in bee venom, melittin, has demonstrated the ability to destroy HIV while preserving normal cells, and has also demonstrated some efficacy against hepatitis and herpes. Before you throw away the condoms, it is important to know that this has just been in the lab, and only when the bee toxin was injected into nanoparticles that poked holes in the outer protective shell of HIV. Don't try this at home, because you couldn't even if you tried.

In other words, if you have some burning or stinging down there, don't think you can simply cure this by sitting on a beehive. If you *do* try this method and get stung repeatedly, assuming you don't immediately die, there are various cures for the allergic reaction. Beyond the standard treatments of allergic reactions with antihistamines and steroids, we bet someone somewhere is investigating herpes as a cure for bee stings.

9

You Can't Redo Everything

As if the birthing process weren't painful enough the first time around, a controversial therapy called "rebirthing therapy" or "attachment therapy" reenacts the birthing process for children who have already been born but who have significant behavioral issues. Some "therapists" have used this extremely controversial practice to treat children with reactive attachment disorder, a condition in which children do not develop healthy, secure attachments or bonds with others. Reactive attachment disorder is rare, but it can result from significant neglect or trauma.

The "rebirthing" involves re-creating the womb, potentially with pillows and blankets. Other details of birth are also simulated, minus any bodily fluids and the placenta. (See: "Placenta: It's Not Just for Breakfast Anymore.") Physical pressure against the child is used to re-create the contractions. The child is to emerge from this experience into the arms of the caregivers to show that they are there to truly embrace and care for the child, kind of like that really aggressive hug your great-aunt used to give.

Considering that these children have not formed good attachments with their caregivers, we're not sure that having the children fight to escape a mock womb would improve that relationship.

But one member of the Association of Rebirthers and Trainers International—you can find a group for everything these days!—clarified that such a re-creation of birth is "birth regression." The member noted that "rebirthing" actually involves a pattern of breathing used over multiple therapy sessions, typically with adults. Some of these adults have claimed that this breathing-with-pillows-and-blankets technique has enabled them to reexperience their own births, or make a really cool fort.

Phew! For a second there we were starting to doubt the validity of "rebirthing," but reexperiencing your own birth while breathing in definitely seems more legitimate than having someone push you with pillows and blankets to re-create your birth.

But that's not a high bar. . . .

10

Country Music Can Be Deadly (for White People)

It is not hard to imagine that songs about debt, discord, divorce, drinking, and dead dogs can lead listeners to become depressed. But can country music really increase the suicide rate? The answer is yes, in metropolitan areas, according to Steven Stack and Jim Gundlach in their study "The Effect of Country Music on Suicide."

According to Stack and Gundlach, the music stresses experiences and challenges that the "subculture" of country-music listeners might be facing in their own lives. Per Stack, these recurrent themes in the music "promote audience identification and . . . promote suicide through the reinforcement of preexisting suicidal moods." Interestingly, however, how "Southern" the city was, or the level of poverty, divorce, or gun availability in the area, did not affect the outcome. Stack also reported that the suicide rate increased in the Caucasian population in forty-nine metropolitan areas when country music was given more airtime.

As one reviewer suggested, there might be other variables at play, like another possible driving force behind suicide in urban areas. Also, to test the findings of Stack's study further, one might have trouble getting the necessary permission from the institutional review board, considering the ethics of rounding up suicidal listeners and exposing them to country music to see if they ultimately kill themselves.

The original study was completed in 1992, before the rise of "pop-country" artists like Kenny Chesney, Keith Urban, Toby Keith, and Tim McGraw. Some of their songs are less about divorce and marital discord and more about family, having fun drinking, kids, having fun drinking, cheating on women, and having fun drinking. So how could any of that lead to suicide? Nevertheless, we're not sure whether depression has improved or actually worsened since Stack's study, given the heavy rotation of Taylor Swift songs everywhere.

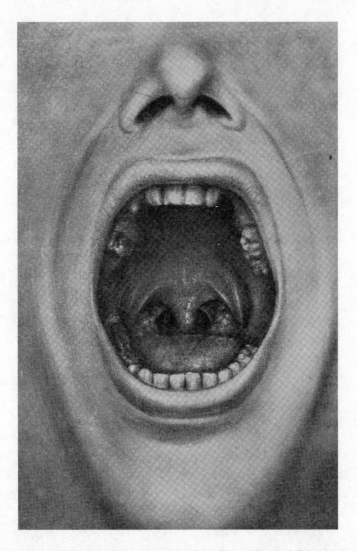

Tooth decay, believed by Henry Cotton to cause mental illness. Obtained from King's College London. As noted on King's College website: Image taken from: Henry A Cotton, MD. *The Defective Delinquent and Insane: The Relation of Focal Infections to Their Causation, Treatment and Prevention.* Princeton: Princeton University Press; London: Oxford University Press, 1921 [IoPHistorical Collection h/Cot].

11

Dark Days: Experimentation on Mentally Challenged and Mentally Ill Patients

In the early 1900s, Dr. Henry Cotton became the director of the New Jersey State Hospital at Trenton, previously called the New Jersey State Lunatic Asylum. We have better names now.

Dr. Cotton's approach to patients was not as soft as his surname suggests. He believed that mental illness was due to infection. Therefore, per Dr. Cotton, whatever body part was infected in a patient must be removed, a practice called "surgical bacteriology."

Dr. Cotton frequently began by extracting patients' teeth, more than eleven thousand in total, according to some accounts, giving both patients and the tooth fairy a lot of pain. If the mental illness persisted, Dr. Cotton, an equal-opportunity remover, employed a sort of "No Organ Left Behind!" mantra and began extracting other organs: gall bladder, spleen, stomach, colon, uterus, ovaries, testicles. Dr. Cotton stayed at the hospital only until 1930, yet teeth extractions remained a practice there until the 1960s, continuing his legacy.

Meanwhile, at the Walter E. Fernald State School in Massachusetts, previously named both the—wait for it—Massachusetts School for Idiotic Children and the—you're welcome—Massachusetts School for the Feeble-Minded, some boys were unaware of the full extent to which they were participating in a Massachusetts Institute of Technology research study. Quaker Oats had given a grant to MIT to study nutrition in the hope that the results would give them a leg up on their rival hot-breakfast manufacturers and maybe, just maybe, solidify Wilford Brimley as their spokesperson while not blaming them for his diabetes.

Told that they were going to be part of a science club, the boys were given oatmeal that contained radioactive tracers, which we hope at least had a Brown Sugar and Cinnamon flavor. A class-action lawsuit in 1995 resulted in Quaker Oats and MIT having to pay money to some of the former Fernald State School residents. Wait, who are the idiotic and feeble-minded ones? We'll never look at the Quaker Oats guy on the can the same way, especially if he seems to be glowing.

Fortunately, in recent decades, federal regulations have been put in place to protect the rights and welfare of what are called "particularly vulnerable populations," including children, pregnant women, prisoners, those who are economically or educationally disadvantaged, and mentally disabled individuals. Just as Wilford Brimley would say about (nonirradiated) oatmeal, "It's the right thing to do, and the tasty way to do it."

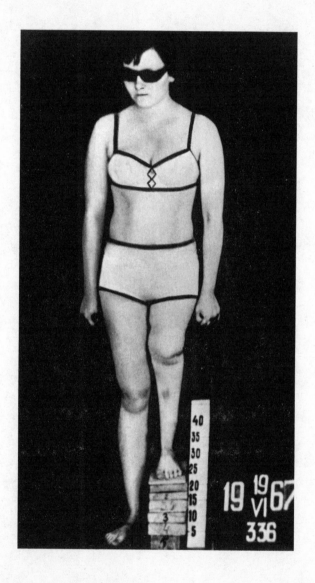

Woman with shortened leg, prior to Iliazarov operation.
Credit: RIA Novosti/Science Source.

12

Stretch Armstrong's Got Nothing on This!

Distraction osteogenesis is not only a pain to write out, but also a surgical procedure used to lengthen the long bones in the body. This might be a treatment option in cases of congenital deformities, or deformities that a person has had since birth, such as different limb lengths or short stature. It has also been used to treat serious traumatic injury. But don't let the name fool you—it is almost impossible to be distracted during this procedure.

Gavriil Abramovich Ilizarov developed a method of distraction osteogenesis, which sounds like something out of *The Texas Chainsaw Massacre* but is actually quite effective and does not involve cannibalism. In the Ilizarov method, an osteotomy, or cut or break in the bone, is made in a way that preserves certain parts of the bone. Then a metal device known as an external fixator, which Ilizarov called the Ilizarov frame—naming it for himself, as most egotistical physicians do—is placed around the limb and screwed into the skin, muscle, and bone. A screw attached to the bone is turned each day to allow a certain amount of distraction, or separation, of the parts of the bone on either side of the osteotomy. This allows new tissue to start growing in between the separated parts of the bone, and over time the bone lengthens. It's almost too easy.

Ilizarov discovered that bone can grow through distraction in 1954 when a patient accidentally distracted the external frame on his leg instead of compressing it. Talk about a boneheaded move, which led decades later to a literally boneheaded move: Ilizarov's principles of distraction have since been applied in cases of micrognathia, or undersized jaw. Such jaw corrections can actually be done in pediatric populations, from newborns to adolescents.

The complications of these procedures can include infection, nerve damage, problems with the devices, and various reactions to anesthesia. We guess you could always opt for no anesthesia, but that might end up looking a lot more like *The Texas Chainsaw Massacre* than you'd like.

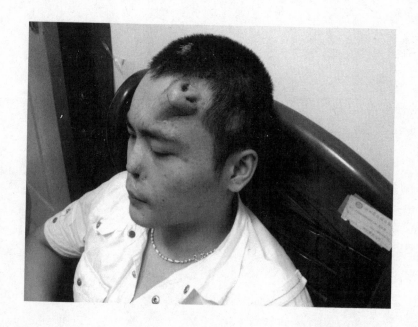

Chinese man, Xiaolian, grows nose on forehead prior to transplant.
Credit: China Stringer Network/Reuters/Landov.

13

Two Eyes, Two Ears, Two Noses?

In 2013, a twenty-two-year-old Chinese man named Xiaolian was revealed to have grown a nose on his forehead. This was not the result of a bizarre, spontaneous second adolescence or the development of an X-Men–like mutation. Surgeons purposely grew the nose on his forehead after Xiaolian had experienced a traumatic injury and an infection that left his existing nose unable to be surgically repaired. Per the explanation by one plastic surgeon, growing a nose on the forehead made sense because the skin of the man's facial area would be more similar to his original nose than if the new nose were grown on another part of his body—say, for example, the back or buttocks. That's one way to avoid ever being called "ass face."

This practice of growing one body part on another part of the body is possible owing to tissue expansion, or the stretching of skin. Plastic surgeons frequently use tissue expansion in cases of restoration, particularly in breast reconstruction after mastectomy. In such cases, an inflatable balloon is placed under the skin, and the skin is stretched. The stretching of the skin causes cellular changes that enable the skin to grow.

In the case of Xiaolian, a tissue expander was used, and then the skin was cut into the shape of a nose. Cartilage from his ribs was later to be transplanted to the proper area of his face to give additional shape to the nose. Such a surgery is not unusual. Tissue is commonly expanded in one site so that it can be later harvested and transplanted to another. This might occur in burn cases, trauma, or other surgical repair. The unusual part of Xiaolian's case was that his nose was formed prior to the transplant.

Growing a nose on a forehead is not nearly the oddest use of tissue transplantation. There are cases in which scrotal tissue has been used for foreskin restoration. Yes, you read that correctly, guys who just crossed your legs. For that ever-so-small population of men who feel that their matadors need their capes back, there is a procedure that details the transplantation of scrotal tissue to the shaft of the penis to re-create the foreskin. Try finding *that* on Pinterest.

For some guys, the idea of this surgery just seems too traumatic. For some women, it may be exactly what their last match.com date needed. Lucky for these guys, there are also nonsurgical methods of foreskin restoration that involve repeated pulling on the penile skin of a circumcised penis for up to twelve hours per day. However, it might take a few years to achieve the form and function that the men are going for. Maybe those guys should talk to Xiaolian's doctors, who would give a whole new meaning to "dick face."

14

I Need This Like I Need a Hole in the Head!

Trepanation, or trephination, is the surgical process of boring a hole in the skull. Today, this is typically, and logically, performed by neurosurgeons who drill a hole to relieve pressure in the brain due to swelling or bleeding or to begin most neurosurgical procedures. Archaeological evidence suggests that in prehistoric and even medieval times, however, you bought yourself a hole in the head if you participated in certain religious ceremonies, joined a particular caste of priests, or were possessed by an evil spirit. And in those days, that hole didn't come easily (that's what she said!); a knifelike instrument was used to scrape away bone or pierce the skull. Consider it the devolved version of "snitches get stitches."

Trepanation was also used as a treatment for mental illness even up to the eighteenth and nineteenth centuries, paving the way for the lobotomy. You'd think that most people who underwent such a procedure did so as a last resort. Well, in 1965, Bart Hughes trepanned himself. Hughes, a big fan of LSD (surprise!) and a former medical student who never graduated (can't imagine why), thought that as human beings evolved to walk, the brain was deprived of the blood that previously supplied it. He argued that by opening up a hole in his head, he could restore the missing blood flow to the brain and also create an everlasting high. Did we mention he liked LSD?

Reports indicate that Hughes took forty-five minutes to trepan himself and then four hours to clean the blood that soaked his apartment. Ten days later, he publicly unveiled his handiwork in a square in Amsterdam, where he unwrapped his head bandages, which read "HA HA HA HA" in multiple colors. Did we mention that he never graduated from medical school—and liked LSD?

Hughes's "operation" influenced others to try the same thing in pursuit of that ultimate high. Years later, Joseph Mellen, who was introduced to Hughes—and consequently LSD—at a party in Ibiza in the 1960s, attempted to trepan himself on multiple occasions to achieve expanded consciousness. Around 1970, Mellen finally succeeded with an electric drill. Per one account, Mellen recalled, "over the next four hours . . . I felt so light and free . . . I felt very relaxed, as if everything would fall into place now." Yeah, that's the feeling of severe blood loss. And this is also what happens when you take advice from a guy who never graduated from medical school, likes LSD, likes to poke holes in his head, and apparently likes to convince other people to try it, too. Worst. Medical. Student. Ever.

15

Asthma, Allergies, and Long-Term Worms

American scientist David Pritchard was searching for a way to tap into the extremely low immune response that Papua New Guineans had when infected by hookworms. Then a not-so-accidental infection with hookworms altered his body chemistry. And now, when David Pritchard grows angry or outraged, a startling metamorphosis occurs. . . . No, Dr. Pritchard does not turn into a giant, verdant, muscular beast, but that sounds less scary than what he did to himself.

Dr. Pritchard did in fact infect himself with hookworms, parasitic worms that have been estimated to kill nearly sixty-five thousand people per year in tropical regions. He did so after he noticed that the people of Papua New Guinea who were infected with hookworms had fewer autoimmune illnesses, like asthma and hay fever. The immune system typically kicks in to attack disease, but in an autoimmune reaction, for some reason your immune system begins to fight against your own body, because sometimes the only thing tough enough to kick your own ass is you.

Dr. Pritchard tried to prove that an infection with hookworms actually decreases autoimmune responses. Lest you think that Dr. Pritchard foolishly dove right into infecting himself, he first asked the people of Papua New Guinea "to collect their fecal matter in buckets for us." He then looked for evidence that the hookworms had actually infected people: hookworm eggs in their stool. Why look there? The hookworm tends to infect people through skin contact, then hitches a ride through the bloodstream to the host's heart and lungs, gets coughed up into the throat, is swallowed, and then hooks itself into the host's gastrointestinal system. As it sucks up the host's blood, it lays plenty of eggs, which are then expelled into the host's feces. Someone walks on the feces, gets the eggs on their skin, and poof—just like that—a new batch of worms finds a new host. It's like poo magic, minus the magic. At least Dr. P. stuck a bandage of worms on himself and skipped skipping in other people's poop.

Given the findings that hookworms diminish hay fever and asthma, some doctors suggest that hookworm infection can help with other autoimmune diseases. People with celiac disease and gluten intolerance, for example, cannot consume gluten in their diet without risking significant stomach upset and excessive flatulence. If they infect themselves with hookworms, that gluten-induced stomach inflammation might just go down. The only problem is that they risk the potential side effects of hookworm infection: significant stomach upset, excessive flatulence, and an embarrassingly extensive trip to the Barnes & Noble bathroom. But for doughnuts and chocolate cake, it would be worth a shot, right?

16

The G-Spot Shot:
Spot On or Spot Off?

The elusive G-spot: not just a rapper anymore. Some women swear they have one, some women swear they don't, and most men just swear repeatedly—and loudly—as they try to find the damn thing. They might have reason to swear; some doctors think the G-spot does not even exist.

Before we go further, let us say that when we were researching this book, for some reason Germans kept coming up—a lot. We have no idea why and have nothing against Germany. We are going to assume the best and say that something in Germany must create a culture of medical innovation, because we like that explanation better than Germany creating a culture of deviance or having fewer safeguards about what you can do to whom. Either way, from here on, feel free to count the unusually high number of references to Germans.

Back to the G-spot. In an article that he wrote in 1950, German gynecologist Ernst Gräfenberg described an erogenous zone "on the anterior [front] wall of the vagina along the course of the urethra [the tubelike structure that carries urine from the bladder to the outside world]."

But the G-doc did not call this the G-spot. He also did not say that stimulation of the area resulted in orgasms—mind-blowing or otherwise. He did say that some women he studied derived orgasm from stimulation of the urethra itself—and those women used hair-pins to do so.

Nearly thirty years after Gräfenberg's article, a group of medical professionals described the case of a woman who found a sensitive area along the anterior wall of her vagina. The group also notes that this woman had the equivalent of a "female ejaculation" when this spot, near the area that Gräfenberg described, hence the "G-spot," was stimulated. As another group later pointed out, how-ever, this woman also had trouble with her bladder falling into her vagina. So who knows exactly what was being stimulated.

Despite the mired and mythological nature of the G-spot, some gynecologists offer G-spot amplification. These physicians have in-jected proteins or polysaccharides found in human connective tis-sue, now in some health and skin-care products (lucky you), into the area between the bladder and the vagina along the anterior vaginal wall. The goals are to make this area larger and more sensitive to stimulation when the penis or any object—hello, hairpins—rubs against it.

One potential concern: Gräfenberg indicated that the sensitive area was on the anterior wall between the vaginal opening and the urethra, not between the bladder and the vagina. So some women might have been getting amplified in the wrong place. Second po-tential concern: It is unclear whether the G-spot actually exists. So what the hell are these women and doctors doing? Wouldn't it just be so much easier and cheaper to go get some hairpins?

17

Chakra the Monkey Tonight!

For thousands of years, Hindu and yogic healers' traditions have described chakras, or wheels of energy, throughout the body. Western interpretation of this ancient belief tells of seven main chakras located in a column from the base of the spine to the head. According to New Age teachings (i.e., anything Californians believe), each of those chakras is associated with a color, and the hue of the colors can vary, depending on a person's emotional, spiritual, and physical state. Consider these chakras a sort of mood ring.

The ancient traditions teach that each chakra contains nerves and organs. If there is a "blockage" in a chakra, energy does not flow well, and there can be subsequent physical or emotional trouble. For example, physical problems resulting from an imbalance in the first chakra can affect the feet, legs, tailbone, rectum, male reproductive organs, and immune system. If you experience constipation, you might have a blockage in this chakra. On the other hand, a Western-medicine doctor might tell you that you have a blockage in your intestine, and it's time to eat some fiber.

Tomato, tomahto.

Some chakra-balancing techniques include yoga, meditation, guided visualization, and reiki, a type of healing by which energy travels into a patient through the hands of the practitioner. In some cases the reiki healer places his hands lightly on the patient, and in other cases the healer holds his hands above the patient. In the case of the hokey pokey, you'll want to put the left hand in. The method is up to the practitioner. So just beware, gentlemen. If you tell your wife your imbalanced chakras are causing sexual dysfunction and she should give you a reiki genital massage, you might get even more sexually frustrated if she opts for a hands-off hand job.

Another treatment for balancing the chakras to restore physical and emotional health is to "eat the rainbow." Before you go digging into a box of Lucky Charms, this refers to eating foods that restore balance based on their colors and what those colors can do for your emotional health. For example, red foods are said to improve energy, yellow foods are said to improve mood, orange bolster confidence, and green impact overall vital energy. Can your Lucky Charms do *that*?

18

Moxibustion: Not Quite Smoking Banana Leaves, but Almost!

In Chinese, Tibetan, and other traditional Asian medical practices, the burning of leaves, or moxibustion, is used to treat various conditions, including facial paralysis. Western medicine teaches that a virus causes some types of facial paralysis, but traditional Chinese medicine suggests that the paralysis occurs when a person's qi (pronounced "chee"), or life force, is frozen by cold air. No wonder none of the Buffalo professional sports teams have ever won a championship.

To treat the frigid qi, some traditional Chinese and Tibetan doctors stimulate acupressure points (acupoints), points on the body that can stimulate the meridians, or anatomic locations through which vital energy flows. In moxibustion, the smoke from a burning packet of moxa, or herbs and leaves, stimulates those acupoints. Mugwort, also known as Saint John's wort, and wormwood, a plant with leaves used in making absinthe, comprise the moxa—it's the closest to Harry Potter names as these things can get. . . .

In direct moxibustion, those leaves burn directly on the skin of the patient at the acupoint location. Maybe your paralysis will resolve, but you have to wonder whether the scarring and pain are worth it. Indirect moxibustion, on the other hand, places moxa above the skin, sometimes on top of garlic or ginger, where they are lit and unfortunately not pan-seared with halibut. In other indirect moxibustion cases the healer ties the moxa to an acupuncture needle that is left in place. If you're having trouble picturing this, just imagine Yosemite Sam after Bugs Bunny has pissed him off—with smoke coming out of his ears.

Moxibustion can in fact treat more than just facial paralysis. No, San Franciscans, you can't smoke it. But a study in the 1990s showed that the process might actually help breech fetuses, or those that are presenting bottom-first, correct their positioning to head-first in the uterus. A 2010 review noted that moxibustion can actually help reduce the nausea and vomiting associated with chemotherapy. Furthermore, moxibustion—hopefully the indirect style—is also said to increase circulation to the pelvis. This doesn't come as too big a surprise, does it? After all, wouldn't anything lit on fire and placed near your pelvis make your blood pump faster?

19

Maybe They Just Passed Gas

For many religious folks, the physical body is merely a vessel for the soul, which lives on after death of the physical form. This belief is based in faith, meaning that scientific evidence does not exist to prove the idea as true or false. However, this doesn't mean that scientists haven't tried to prove such ideas.

In the early 1900s, Massachusetts physician Duncan McDougall set out to determine that the human soul had mass and was therefore scientifically measurable. He gathered six humans, each in the final stages of death, and closely watched them in individual beds that were each located on one side of a balancing scale—the way most of us would choose to go. The scales were designed specifically for Dr. McDougall's experiment and were sensitive to weight within one-tenth of an ounce. Reports indicate that Dr. McDougall monitored each person and calculated their weight loss in the final hours of death. He considered that some of the final weight loss could be due to evaporation of sweat and moisture from breathing. However, upon the exact moment of their death or one minute later, Dr. McDougall noted that a significant change in weight occurred in four of the six individuals before him. He blamed mechanical failures and the experiment not being set up completely in the other two cases.

Dr. McDougall found that one individual lost approximately twenty-one grams at death. In order to prove that this was not due to the body's final exhaling of air, Dr. McDougall got on the scale himself and forcefully exhaled to try to create a change in weight. He couldn't make the scale budge. In a later experiment, he took fifteen dogs in their final moments of death—no PETA back then, clearly—and tried to re-create his experiment. He found no change in weight, which he took to mean that the human soul definitively had a weight. You might be skeptical or surprised by this mass of twenty-one grams—after all, who uses the metric system?!

Although fascinating, Dr. McDougall's work likely does not stand up to modern scientific scrutiny and standards of precision. His results varied between patients, with some losing half an ounce, per his records, and others more than that. When the final moment of death occurred was unclear, and two people could not be included in the work because of scientific or human error. So, not a huge body of evidence to suggest that this is scientific proof of the soul having mass and existence.

One of the most interesting moments in Dr. McDougall's experiments occurred when one of the six patients died and there was no immediate change in weight. Oh, those stubborn pounds after death. After one minute, however, there was a change in weight. He explained, "I believe that in this case, that of a phlegmatic man slow of thought and action, that the soul remained suspended in the body after death, during the minute that elapsed before its freedom. There is no other way of accounting for it, and it is what might be expected to happen in a man of the subject's temperament." In other words, if you are a sluggish person in real life, your soul is just as sluggish in the afterlife.

Dr. McDougall's follow-up "scientific studies" might make some question his work even more. He claimed that the soul should be visible on an X-ray because "at the moment of death the soul substance might become so agitated as to reduce the obstruction that the bone of the skull offers ordinarily to the Roentgen ray [X-ray] and might therefore be shown on the plate as a lighter spot on the dark shadow of the bone." He then spent time trying to photograph the soul leaving the body at the moment of death. It is unknown whether he lost twenty-one grams or showed a "lighter spot" on an X-ray upon his own death, in 1920.

20

As If Birth Weren't Traumatic Enough

Anyone who has witnessed the birth of a child, or at least watched it on Lifetime, can tell you that the mother appears to be in a great amount of pain. Typically, the mother, and everyone around her, would like to do anything possible to reduce that pain or comfort the mother.

Enter the water birth. Literally. And unlike when most people use the word "literally," we truly mean "literally."

A water birth typically involves the mother sitting in a warm bath so that she and her as-yet-unborn baby are immersed in water during labor. Some evidence suggests that immersion in water does decrease pain, the use of anesthesia, and the duration of labor during the first stage of labor. This first stage lasts until the cervix is fully dilated. Then the second stage of labor begins, during which the mother has to push the baby out into the world.

Some mothers exit the bath after the first stage of labor, while others remain in the water for the actual birth. Some feel like this is a more natural transition to life, or they want to be in their homes and have the flexibility to move around in a warm bath. Sure, this sounds very kale, Birkenstock, and Zen, but evidence is lacking to support that the baby or mother has a better outcome if immersed in water during the second stage of labor. In fact, some serious side effects, although rare, can occur during that second stage of labor, such as: higher risk of infection for the mother and baby, the baby breathing in tub water and potentially drowning or nearly drowning, and umbilical-cord rupture as the newborn is maneuvered out of the tub. The American College of Obstetricians and Gynecologists (ACOG) has therefore stated, "The practice of immersion in the second stage of labor (underwater delivery) should be considered an experimental procedure that only should be performed within the context of an appropriately designed clinical trial with informed consent."

Some might scoff at this and say that an entry into the world through warm water is still better for the child. Better how, exactly? It's not as if the child is going to remember the birth and thank you later—although, it wouldn't kill you to do that, Zachary. We are also not aware of studies that show greater self-soothing ability, success, or morality in those who experienced a water birth. So maybe hang on before you go purchasing those pool noodles.

One water birth website posts, "The women who have experienced the support and comfort of water for their labors and held their newborns in their arms speak more than any scientific article or paper on the subject." We're not quite sure, but we think ACOG might disagree—as might every scientist and doctor in the world, or anyone else who went to school and studied the human body for a minimum of nine years.

21

An Eerie Enema

Arnold Ehret, the author of *The Definitive Cure of Chronic Consti-pation*, reportedly said, "Life is a tragedy of nutrition." Well, it turns out, sometimes life is also a (rather disturbing) comedy when it comes to treating constipation. A case in point is a patient reported in the journal *Surgery* in 2004, who attempted to use an eel to treat his constipation.

Stay with us here.

Now, the idea of eating eels to cure constipation is not new, and many have held this belief, especially in the traditional Danish cul-ture. The rationale behind this belief is not clear. Eels do have a reputation for being "slippery," so maybe some think the eels' slip-periness will help evacuate the bowels.

However, the case mentioned in *Surgery* is a bit different: it in-volves inserting the eel into the *other* end, i.e., the anus, to treat constipation. The patient, a fifty-year-old male, presented to the emergency department with the complaint of abdominal pain. An X-ray of his abdomen showed the outline of an eel, and upon fur-ther questioning, the patient admitted to inserting the eel to relieve constipation. The patient required an emergency surgery, and doc-tors found and removed a nearly twenty-inch eel. The eel had bitten part of the patient's bowel, resulting in an inch-long perforation (tear). Fortunately, the surgeons were able to repair the damage, and the patient was discharged home after about a week. The authors end by saying, "This may be related to a bizarre health care belief, inadvertent sexual behavior, or criminal assault. However, the true reason may never be known."

Whatever the reason, at the risk of seeming too practical, may we recommend treating constipation with more fiber in the diet instead of an elongated fish up the bum? Remember, kale doubles as nature's Shop-Vac.

Beyond that, in this case it's hard to know who to feel more sorry for, the eel or the man; both were probably shocked in the end (heyoh!).

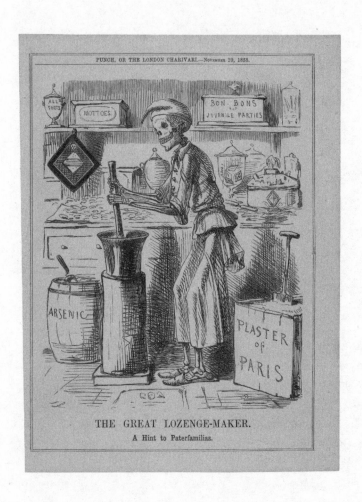

A not-so-subtle image hinting at the fate of consuming arsenic-laden products.
Credit, as listed on Wikipedia: John Leech (caricaturist) (1817–1864). First published in *Punch* (London), 20 November 1858. Public domain.

22

They Say Stripes Are Slimming

Arsenic. Atomic number 33. This bad boy really can do bad things, in both the Michael Jackson bad cool way and the bad terrible way, like Justin Bieber songs.

Arsenic has existed for over three thousand years and was added to bronze during the Bronze Age to make the metal harder. That's not the only thing it made harder over the years. In the 1850s, some men in a remote area of Austria swallowed bits of arsenic to improve their libido. Women who swallowed small chunks of the element had a rosier complexion, likely due to increased blood flow caused by the arsenic. This led to the production of beauty products, such as soaps and skin applications, that contained arsenic. It was also used in certain green and purple dyes over the years.

The only problem: Arsenic is very toxic and can be fatal. In fact, arsenic is so deadly when ingested in large enough quantities that it has been referred to as "inheritance powder."

When a person ingests too much arsenic, his breath and bodily fluids, such as urine, might smell like garlic. The person might experience an increased heart rate, decreased blood pressure, altered mental status, diarrhea, coma, and seizures. Fingernails might show wide striped bands, which are called Mees' lines, and might look pretty cool if not for the fact that they indicate that someone has arsenic poisoning.

One example of large-scale arsenic poisoning occurred in 1858, in Bradford, England. There, a man known as Humbug Billy sold striped, hard-boiled candies called humbugs, which—the story tells—Billy bought from a man named Neal. According to the story, Neal did not want to pay the expensive fees for sugar, so Neal would cut the candy ingredients, as one might cut cocaine, with a substitute that he got from the pharmacy. That substitute was not always comprised of the highest-quality, organic, grass-fed, free-range ingredients. As you guessed, Neal once made a batch with arsenic that the pharmacist mistakenly provided, and Humbug Billy then sold that batch. Around two hundred people became sick and nearly twenty died. Not surprising, considering how bad English food is, even without the arsenic.

Physicians have harnessed arsenic for good use recently, using arsenic trioxide, a manufactured form of arsenic, to treat patients with some types of leukemia. Arsenic trioxide has been shown to help reduce remission rates in a large percentage of patients with acute promyelocytic leukemia, a type of blood cancer. And for those who want to experiment with mummification a bit, arsenic poisoning does a great job of preserving a body. The element not only kills the body's cells, but it also kills any bacteria that would break down the body. So you actually *can* live fast, die young, and leave a good-looking corpse. You just need to be poisoned to do it. Small price.

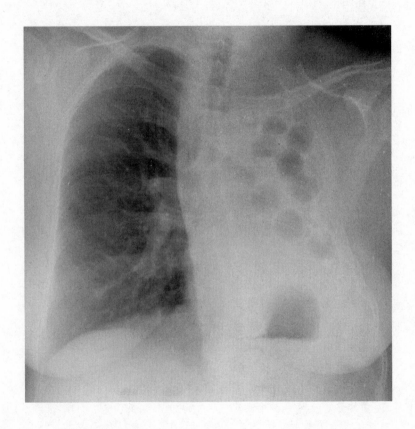

X-ray showing the outline of lucite spheres used to collapse a patient's lung.
Credit: Case courtesy of Dr. David Clemo Steel, Radiopaedia.org, rID: 35019
(image owned by Radiopaedia).

23

Ping-Pong, Anyone?

Tuberculosis (TB) is an infectious disease that spreads through the air when people with an active TB infection cough, sneeze, talk, or transmit into the air secretions associated with breathing. Once the leading cause of death in the United States, TB most often infects the lungs. Prior to the development and use of the proper medications to treat TB in the 1950s, physicians treated the disease by trying to collapse the infected part of the lung. The idea was that the infected part of the lung would heal faster if it was collapsed.

Interesting idea, but how do you collapse someone's lung?

You have to introduce air into the space between the inside of the chest wall and the outside of the lung, called the pleural cavity. Before physicians had drugs to treat TB, they would inject air into the pleural space to collapse the lung, but then they would have to reinject air repeatedly to keep the lung collapsed. They then developed a method of collapsing the lung called plombage.

Plombage involved inserting objects, called plombs, into the pleural space so that the lung would remain collapsed. The objects used as plombs included: fat; oil; plastic sponges; solid paraffin wax, an ingredient in making candles and sometimes chocolate candies to help them harden with a sheen; and Lucite (transparent plastic) balls that were similar in size and shape to Ping-Pong balls. The development of anti-TB drugs made this practice almost obsolete.

It's a good thing, because complications of this procedure have included infection, fistulas (abnormal connections between organs or structures in the body), erosion of blood vessels, cancers associated with the material makeup of the plombs, and a strong desire to play table tennis.

At times radiologists do see evidence of plombage on imaging, typically in older patients who were treated for TB back before the 1950s. Dark, circular shapes appear on the imaging in the lung area, typically indicating the presence of the Lucite balls. On occasion, these plombs do need to be removed. In a case report from 2009, an eighty-year-old man complained of a fever and swelling along his front left shoulder area that was increasing in size and preventing him from moving his neck fully. Surgeons found and removed sheets of plastic and twenty-three Lucite balls, mostly filled with pus, that were initially placed in the patient's chest (pus-free) fifty-nine years earlier. He recovered well, according to the report.

Did that eighty-year-old have balls or what?

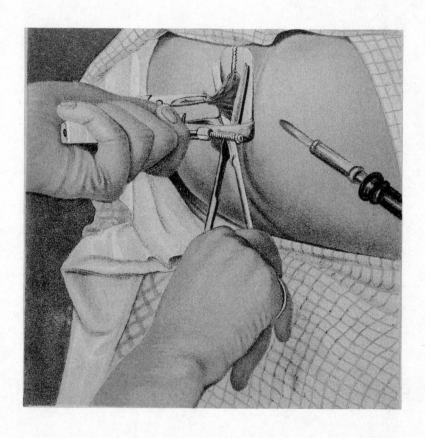

Internal hemmorhoid clamped, about to be cut and cauterized. Image from page 530 of *Diseases of the Rectum and Anus: Designed for Students and Practitioners of Medicine* (1910) by Samuel Goodwin Gant. Public Domain.

24

Treating Hemorrhoids:
A Real Pain in the Butt

Hemorrhoids. Those unsexy, clumpy, inflamed veins around or inside the anus that can bleed, itch, or generally just make you feel not-so-fresh each time you try to move your bowels. Hemorrhoids occur when the veins around the anus are inflamed, or whenever Ke$ha puts out a new single. This typically happens more frequently for women during pregnancy, and for everyone as the aging process occurs. Other reasons for the irritation of hemorrhoids include: chronic diarrhea or chronic constipation, straining during bowel movements, sitting for long periods on the toilet, and anal intercourse. So be warned! Spend less time on the toilet playing Candy Crush and maybe reconsider whether an intimate entrance up your exit ramp is a good idea.

Nearly four-fifths of North American and European adults experience hemorrhoids, men more than women. Overall, hemorrhoids can be awful—but not as awful as some of the treatments for them throughout history have been.

Egyptian writings indicate that a concoction of ground and cooked acacia leaves smeared on a strip of linen would immediately relieve hemorrhoids—if a person inserted said soaked linen into his anus. Hippocrates apparently suggested tying off the hemorrhoids with a needle and thread and then applying hellebore, a poisonous plant, to the area after some time. If we had a quarter for every time someone told us to do that . . . But the most painful method appears to be the medieval manner of treatment: cauterizing the hemorrhoids with a hot iron or cutting into them with a sharp knife—not exactly *Grey's Anatomy* plot fodder. In fact, medieval illustrations depicting the performance of such procedures show a steady stream of blood pouring down from the anus of the patient. If surgery is needed today, it is much more civilized and typically occurs after numerous other, more tame measures, such as treatment with creams, ointments, ice, or warm baths, have not shown results.

Back in medieval times, people did have an option if they really wanted to try something noninvasive to treat hemorrhoids: prayer to Saint Fiacre, the Irish patron saint of hemorrhoids. As the story goes, the local bishop offered Fiacre, who also became the patron saint of gardeners, as much land as he could cultivate in one day. Using only a small spade, he presumably spent a long time squatting during those twenty-four hours and ultimately developed some pretty atrocious hemorrhoids. Legend says that he sat on a stone, prayed for relief, and was cured.

The stone is now called Saint Fiacre's stone, and some say it shows the imprints of Saint Fiacre's hemorrhoids. Apparently people still travel to the stone to pray for the amazing cure Saint Fiacre experienced. We just hope Saint Fiacre's stone is not like the Blarney Stone, which you're supposed to kiss in order to harness its power.

25

Sore Throat: Better or Worse After These Remedies?

The cause of a sore throat is typically a viral infection. The same way that a virus causes the body aches of the flu, it can cause the discomfort of a sore throat, a runny nose, and congestion. Although many aching patients ask their physicians for antibiotics, antibiotics treat bacterial infections and not viral infections. Usually it's just a matter of waiting out the virus and managing the symptoms. However, that never stops people from trying homemade remedies, like gargling salt water, drinking hot water, or applying processed animal parts or by-products directly to the neck. Although, we'd never turn down a good filet mignon wrap, if that were a thing. Is it a thing?

In the 1898 book *Essential Lessons in Human Physiology and Hygiene for Schools*, Winfred E. Baldwin notes that there are many types of sore throat, some of which can be "very serious." Baldwin states that because of this, "[I]t is always advisable that a physician should be consulted." The author's modern-day insight seems to end there. The author next reports that applying lard, Vaseline, or salt pork to a piece of flannel and then attaching it to the throat would be helpful in recovery from the sore throat.

Utah folk medicine offers even more pork products as potential treatments. One antidote involved tying a strip of fresh bacon around the neck with a dirty sock or, in the case of a child having a sore throat, putting black pepper on bacon and putting the peppered end against the neck. We're not quite sure why that is particularly helpful for a child—or anyone for that matter. Some remedies suggested applying carrots and onions to a paper or cloth around the neck. Seems odd, but at least you'd have the start of a decent stew. At any rate, it's still more appealing than placing chicken droppings in a cloth and tying it around the neck, as one treatment called for.

More unusual than these vegetable- and swine-laden curative measures are those that involved kerosene. (Bacon neck doesn't sound so bad now, does it?) As Elisabeth Janos details in her work *Country Folk Medicine*, some people added a few drops of kerosene to a teaspoon of sugar and swallowed it down to relieve the pain in the throat. Clearly these details were omitted from the original Mary Poppins version of the song.

The use of kerosene didn't stop there. Some people gargled it to combat their sore throats, despite its taste. Other people applied kerosene to the outside of the throat. In fact, one person described his experience having a kerosene-soaked rag placed around his neck by his mother: "The sore throat went right away, but I had a mess of blisters." Imagine that.

Clearly Child Protective Services didn't often visit the place where that happened, and neither will we, hopefully.

26

Facing the Facts When, in Fact, That's Not Your Face

Modern medical doctors really can perform miraculous transformations. No, we're not talking about breast implants. We're talking about giving people with severely disfigured faces the chance to actually feel more comfortable with themselves and to improve their overall mental and physical health. How? By means of a face transplant.

Although this sounds like something out of a horror movie, the procedure has actually been successfully completed multiple times, not counting in the John Travolta 1997 cinematic masterpiece *Face/Off*. In 2005, surgeons in northern France performed the first partial face transplant on Isabelle Dinoire, whose own dog brutally attacked her. The physicians transplanted the nose, chin, and lips, including the skin, soft tissue, and muscle, from a donor face to the patient's mauled face. Using microvascular surgical techniques, the doctors connected blood vessels and nerves from the transplanted facial region to those remaining on Ms. Dinoire's face. She admitted that she was scared to look at herself after the procedure, but remarked that when she did she found the face "beautiful."

In March 2012, an extensive medical team comprised of more than 150 nurses and professional staff, with additional trauma, plastic and reconstructive, and maxillofacial surgeons at the University of Maryland Medical Center's R Adams Cowley Shock Trauma Center, completed a full face transplant on a man who had suffered a severe gunshot wound to his face more than ten years earlier. The family of an anonymous organ donor donated the face, including the tongue, teeth, and upper and lower jaws. The transplant took one and a half days and involved surgical procedures on skin, tissue, muscles, nerves, and bone. The end goal was to transplant and shape a fully functioning face that could sense touch and express emotion. Pictures from June 2013 suggest that this is exactly what the team accomplished.

Following face transplants, the recipients must take medicines to lower their immune system's likelihood of rejecting the new face. In some cases, the medications themselves can have side effects, including increased cancer risks. It seems like the potential for these side effects might pale in comparison to the trauma that these individuals have endured. Some of the people who have undergone face transplants have experienced such horrific incidents as: savage mauling from dogs, bears, and chimpanzees; car accidents; shotgun blasts; the physical beating from a spouse who then threw lye on his wife's face; and severe burns from a high-voltage electrical line.

As Dr. Eduardo Rodriguez at the University of Maryland reminds us, it is an amazing gift that someone would donate her face so that someone else can have it. In fact, that seems to be the most remarkable aspect of the face transplant: not that modern medicine can make it to happen, but that someone else—a complete stranger to the recipient—can.

27

Stocks Drop, So Might the Bodies

Money does funny things to people. Some come into money and become more philanthropic. Others become more selfish and greedy. Still others don't let it affect them at all. But when it comes to losing money, it's hard not to be affected in some way. Anecdotal evidence of your friendly neighborhood stockbroker getting sad and crying is one thing, but recent studies by financial professors and medical doctors have shown us that when the stock market tanks, so does our physical and mental health.

Finance professors Joseph Engelberg and Christopher A. Parsons reported that on Black Monday (October 19, 1987), when stock prices dove 25 percent, hospital admissions in California increased by 5 percent. The professorial duo noted that an increase in hospital admissions for mental-health issues, such as anxiety, panic attacks, and major depression, occurred on the very same day that the stocks crashed. This suggests a strong link between psychological health and stock-portfolio health.

And what about physical health? A group from Duke University reviewed 11,590 cases of patients hospitalized in the local area during a time of stock-market decrease in value between October 2008 and April 2009. The authors of the study noted "significant correlation between a period of stock market decrease and increased" rates of heart attack.

So are we really at the mercy of our finances?

Possibly. It is impossible to know whether every person in these studies admitted to the hospital for mental-health issues or a heart attack actually had a vested interest in the stock market or even owned stocks. But the trend of hospitalizations for these issues did suddenly change at a time of financial volatility, suggesting that the link is there.

Did we really need studies telling us this, though? After all, the entire decade following the stock-market crash of October 1929 was called the Great Depression. This is true, but the immediacy of the effect a significant downturn in the stock market has on the psyche, occurring in the same day, and not just sometime over a decade, gives us an important insight into this powerful link.

Yikes. Maybe Trent Reznor was right when he wrote and ~~sang~~ screamed "Head Like a Hole."

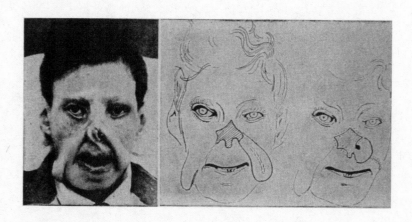

Pedicle graft (*left*) with illustration showing process of converting left side into a nose, (*right*). Image from page 1273 of *Manual of Operative Surgery* (1921) by John Fairbairn Binnie. Public Domain.

28

It's Just a Flesh Wound

One of the longest surgeries one of us witnessed during medical school was a seventeen-hour transfer of tissue from the leg of a patient to her mouth. The patient required reconstruction of her tongue and jaw, which had been invaded by cancer. Aside from contaminating himself five times during that case, getting yelled at by the surgical nurses, and realizing he never wanted to see another operating room in his life, the author learned that the skin taken from the leg and then moved to the patient's mouth was called a free flap or free-tissue transfer.

Free flaps are sections of tissue, such as skin, fat, muscle, or bone, with their arteries and veins, detached completely from one area of the body and reattached, with their blood vessels, to another part of the body. These "flaps" are considered "free" because they are completely transferred. The predecessor to this type of tissue transfer was called the pedicle graft, or walking skin graft. This was definitely not free by any means.

New Zealand–born plastic surgeon Sir Archibald McIndoe created walking skin grafts, which were tubelike structures of fat and skin connecting the tissue-donation site on the body and the site where the tissue would be transferred. Gradually Dr. McIndoe "walked" the tissue to its new location in a series of operations in which he would reattach the donation end to sites closer and closer to the receiving end needing the tissue. Eventually, he would walk the tissue to its final destination, having kept it alive the whole time. Dr. Harold Gillies used a similar tubed pedicle method and swung a flap of skin from the patient's chest or forehead over the patient's face. No big deal.

Pretty brilliant, but pretty horrific in appearance. Think of the face huggers from *Alien* or the long tubes on the side of the head of Predator. Or shepherd's pie. But despite their unappetizing look, the tubed pedicles kept the tissue alive at a time when doctors did not have the antibiotics necessary to preserve the tissue and treat infection.

And while those grafts might have looked strange, they're nothing compared with some of the oddities one might see when a free flap from another part of the body is moved to the mouth to reconstruct the oral area after cancer. Sometimes patients wind up with part of a tattoo on their new tongue, or even hair growth after a section of the leg or arm is moved to the mouth. Talk about a hairball!

29

When Blood Is Green
and Urine Blue

When blood cells carry oxygen, the blood is red. Generally, we expect blood to be red, but in fact, it's a bit blue inside most of our veins because the blood has been delivered to the organs that take out the oxygen they need. The deoxygenated blood then travels back to the lungs and soaks up more oxygen, becoming the familiar red color once again.

So you can imagine how shocked some Canadian physicians were when they found a patient's blood to be a completely different color. While treating a man for severe lower-leg problems, the medical team tried to place a catheter in an artery in his arm. The blood came back a greenish-black color. We'll let you insert the requisite Vulcan/Mr. Spock/*Star Trek* joke here yourself.

Upon testing, the team found that the man had been taking a significant dose, perhaps even too much, of the medication sumatriptan, which can treat migraine headaches. In rare cases, the red blood cells in the body incorporate the sulphur atoms of this medication. The result, called sulfhemoglobin, is greenish blood. In this Canadian case, the patient stopped taking his sumatriptan, and his blood appeared red again when doctors saw him five weeks later.

Green blood is surely strange, but how about blue urine? Certain drugs can cause urine to have a bluish color, including methylene blue, which treats carbon-monoxide poisoning, and that little blue pill that has risen (ha!) in popularity in the past two decades: Viagra. Typically the dyes and chemicals in the medications cause the pee to have that chic Windex sheen.

A patient of ours experienced this side effect once and discovered it while attending a major-league baseball game. After a few highly overpriced beverages, he went to the men's room and found himself a spot at the end of the trough urinal. As he began relieving himself, he noticed a blue stream heading down the trough. He wasn't the only one who noticed: the other ten men at the urinal, breaking traditional urinal etiquette, stopped looking straight ahead and immediately looked directly at him. The patient was quite embarrassed, apologized to everyone, and said on his way out, "I'm a really big Michigan fan. Go Blue or go home!"

30

Prosthetic Limbs of Today: Beyond Pegs and Hooks

A prosthetic limb is an artificial limb that substitutes for the missing body part. Over the years, researchers, engineers, and scientists have made significant strides in both the appearance and function of prostheses. Compare Mr. Han and his hook hand in Bruce Lee's *Enter the Dragon* with the rubbery look of the one-armed man in *The Fugitive* and with the more technical hand replacement of Luke Skywalker in *The Empire Strikes Back*. Although these are on-screen characters, the fictional depiction of prosthetic arms and hands parallels the detailed, realistic changes over the years. This amazing evolution was highly welcomed, especially considering the unwanted side effects of some of the earlier prosthetics.

Consider some of the joint replacements in the 1970s. (No, not *those* joints.) Some of the metal, plastics, and bone cement that were used in certain types of prosthetic joints on occasion included cobalt and chromium. According to some studies in animals, these elements could cause the development of tumors. In the case of one sixty-six-year-old man, the patient had inflammation of the skin where he had a joint replacement, and testing showed that it was related to exposure to cobalt.

Modern-day prosthetic joints and limbs can still cause some complications, as can any surgery and introduction of a foreign material into the human body. But the materials and the look of the prosthetics are quite nuanced. Silicone gels that allow a more comfortable fit have replaced some of the hard plastics once used. More recently, a feedback system has been developed to allow a patient with a below-the-knee amputation to "feel" the limb. The system involves the inflation of balloons when a patient walks using his prosthetic leg. The pressure from those balloons is felt on the patient's thigh and lets him know whether he is properly balancing himself on his prosthetic foot. We're sure the Sea Captain from *The Simpsons* is quite envious.

It seems that not all patients would appreciate the technologically savvy, modern-day prostheses. Take, for example, the case of a man in Florida in 2013 who was in a car that police pulled over for missing a taillight. Police first asked the passengers if they had any drugs or weapons in the car, to which they replied, "No." Upon noticing the man's prosthetic leg, police asked him if he had any drugs in his prosthetic leg. The man seemingly folded easily, because he then handed over a bag of cocaine. (Of note: The female driver then removed morphine and hydromorphone from her bra and a hypodermic needle from her buttocks.)

Similarly, in Massachusetts, police pulled over a woman for having overly tinted windows. Upon finding drugs in her possession, the police patted her down and found that her buttocks seemed particularly hard.

Her first excuse? "I don't have a butt," she stated. Continuing with, "I wear these [underwear] and another pair of underwear under it." Exercising their keen intuition, the police asked her to remove the fake butt. Police then found two plastic baggies containing thirteen oxycodone pills altogether and a bag containing $350 of heroin.

Perhaps the people in these cases would benefit best from a prosthetic brain.

31

Want Bigger Breasts? Have a Thai Stranger Slap Them Repeatedly

Some people go to whatever lengths necessary to sculpt their bodies into the most perfect physical specimen possible. Makeup. Exercises. Photoshop. While we've heard of a variety of approaches to shape the shape, we're pretty sure most people haven't tried this one.

A Thai woman named Khemmikka Na Songkhla, more commonly known as Khunying Tobnom and Madame Breastslapper, practices the "art" of breast slapping, as passed down from her grandmother. Oh, there's more. Tobnom reports that when she was a teenager, her grandmother slapped her (Tobnom's) breasts multiple times and then doused them in cold water. Tobnom explained that her breasts grew by four inches after this. It's such a shame that teenagers don't go through a natural growth spurt that makes their bodies grow into more developed adult forms.

Tobnom does not attribute breast growth to puberty at all. Instead, her punching and kneading motions are designed to redistribute fat from places on the body where fat is not desirable to places where it is desired, such as the breast area. But Tobnom does not *just* offer breast slapping (because that would be weird?); she also provides buttock and face punching—for a cost, of course.

Reports from 2013 indicate that she was offering six ten-minute breast-slapping sessions for a total of $380. Some of her protégés in San Francisco charge much steeper prices, however: $1,000 for four face-slapping sessions, which are supposed to improve facial appearance, decrease wrinkles, and even raise eyebrows.

Don't blame Tobnom's students for charging more. They have to make back the money they spent to learn the art directly from Madame Breastslapper. In 2011, she started to teach the procedures to a very select few for approximately $40,000. By 2014, tuition had increased: $350,000 to learn buttock punching, $350,000 to learn face slapping, and $700,000 to learn breast slapping ($350,000 per boob, obviously).

While some of you might question the safety of these methods—and we can't imagine why you wouldn't—don't worry. The Thai Health Ministry conducted a study on women between the ages of twenty and sixty who received breast-slapping and massage treatments over six months. Their results indicated that breast size did increase with no increased risk for cancer.

Phew! We can all breathe a sigh of relief now and feel a lot safer baring our breasts—and faces and buttocks—to people we've never met before so that they can pummel them for several minutes with their hands for hundreds of dollars. Sounds totally worry-free, medically indicated, and legitimate.

32

Truly Giving a Shit

Irked and inflamed by your irritable bowels? Here's one treatment you might not have considered: fecal transplant.

Yes, you read that correctly.

Otherwise known as fecal microbiota transplantation, or FMT, this procedure might be an option for those who have chronic gastrointestinal infection caused by *Clostridium difficile*. *C. diff*, as they are affectionately known, are bacteria that populate and take over the gut when antibiotics have killed the natural, healthy bacteria in the gut. You may remember *C. diff* from the Fox special *When Good Bacteria Turn Bad*.

C. diff infection can lead to chronic diarrhea, inflammation of the colon, or, at its worst, toxic megacolon, which sounds like a reptilian villain from a bad Godzilla movie but is actually a severe distension of the colon that can lead to death if left untreated.

To replace the healthy bacteria, doctors might recommend taking probiotics, or biotics that have left their amateur careers and are now getting paid big bucks. For severe cases, fecal transplantation might be an option. In these cases, the donor fecal matter, with the healthy, natural gut bacteria, can be delivered to a patient infected with *C. diff*. The desired stool can be delivered to a recipient in different ways: via a tube through the nose that leads to the stomach (nasogastric tube); via a tube through the nose to the small intestine (nasojejunal tube); via a tube with a light on it that goes into the mouth, down the esophagus, and deeper into the gastrointestinal tract (endoscopy); and via a tube that goes through the anus and into the colon (colonoscopy). FMT can also be akin to a reverse enema (i.e., when a donor's stool is inserted into the rectum of a patient). While all of these processes sound disgusting, the bacterial repopulation of the colon can lead to remarkable results. One study indicates an average success rate of over 90 percent, making us feel quite badly for the remaining 10 percent.

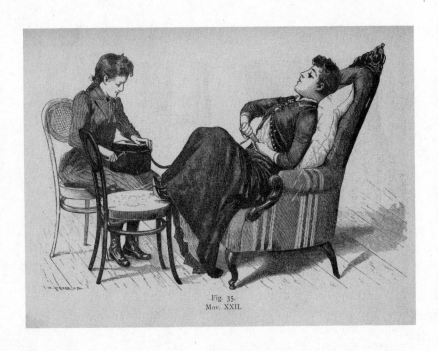

Fig. 35.
Mov. XXII.

Demonstration of the vibrator, a description of the vibrator (Engl. pat. 1890.
No.4390.) and directions for use by C. H. Liedbeck. Credit: Wellcome Library,
London. Obtained from: Creative Commons by 4.0.

33

"Hands-On" Help for Hysteria

We naturally worry in certain situations: public speaking, first dates, breaking and entering. Such anxiety might be protective. That nervous energy can drive us to perform better or make better-informed decisions. Nevertheless, many doctors become concerned when anxiety impairs a patient's daily functioning. Although anxiety can happen in anyone, in centuries past, doctors felt anxiety was a condition in women, and such women were known as "hysterical." This term is not used to describe just women anymore, at least not by men who still want their wives to speak to them.

Some physicians thought that hysteria stemmed from sexual deprivation. Many past treatments for hysteria reflected this theory, as physicians performed pelvic bleeding procedures, surgically removed the ovaries, and even repeated vaginal or "pelvic" massage until these women achieved orgasm to relieve the hysteria—or at least that is why the physicians said they were doing it.

The popularity of the personal vibrator actually has its roots in the latter procedure. We imagine medical malpractice also has its roots here.

34

Kim Kardashian's Vampire Facial (No, Not *That* Kind!)

When you read the term "vampire facial," we know where your mind goes! In reality, what sounds like the end of an Internet porno starring Kim and pale creatures of the night is actually an attempt by some dermatologists to rejuvenate a patient's face.

Also known as a "blood facial," the "vampire facial" is a procedure in which a patient's blood is drawn, placed in vials, and then put in a centrifuge. In the centrifuge—think of that scrambler amusement-park ride, but for test tubes—the blood is spun extremely fast. The heavier parts of the blood sink to the bottom of the tube, and the lighter parts rise to the top. That top layer is full of plasma, the liquid part of blood, and the smaller platelets, which are full of growth factors. This plasma-platelet component is then placed on the patient's face so it can be reabsorbed and aid in the creation of new tissue.

See, completely natural and completely disgusting!

Many celebrities have embraced this procedure, including most prominently Kim Kardashian—although some might think her face is not the only place where "growth factors" have been placed. Given Kim's aptitude for science, particularly molecular-level hematologic function, she must have read and thoroughly enjoyed the 2012 study suggesting that the growth factors found in platelets aided new tissue growth in the skin. To some, the next logical step would be to study this procedure more thoroughly and understand the science. To some dermatologists, the next logical step would be to poke microscopic holes in someone's face and charge around $1,500 for the hope for a brighter, more youthful-looking face.

That online vampire porn video seems slightly less disturbing now, doesn't it?

35

MADW Wasn't Quite as Catchy

As physicians we have seen many consequences of alcohol use, from trauma to liver disease to epic breakups in an Applebee's parking lot. Drunk driving alone causes more than ten thousand deaths per year, almost a third of all driving-related fatalities. While this has deservedly received extensive attention from police and private organizations, apparently an even more dangerous activity runs rampant: drunk walking.

As detailed in *Freakonomics*, an analysis was performed on drunk walking. The basic principle was simple: Take the number of deaths due to walking intoxicated per mile walked, compared with the number of deaths due to driving intoxicated per mile driven. We are not quite sure how the authors collected the data and if that collection method was reliable, but the authors found that the risk of death from drunk walking was eight times that from drunk driving. Based on this logic, if intoxicated, one would be safer driving drunk than walking drunk.

Clearly there's more at play here. First of all, several factors might be skewing the statistics. Typically many more miles are covered when driving compared with walking, so if you were to compare deaths per instance of time walking and deaths per instance of time driving, the comparison wouldn't be nearly as lopsided. In addition, drunk walkers, future characters on *The Walking Dead*, could very well be walking when there are more drunk drivers on the road, increasing walkers' chances of getting hit. Finally, a drunk walker uses an entirely different moral compass when putting himself in danger than does a drunk driver who endangers others. We have humbly suggested to some of our patients that they avoid both situations by simply not drinking at all. Unfortunately, that sounded even crazier to them than drunk driving or drunk walking.

36

A Load of Bully

Because most physical and mental health problems take a long time to progress, they do not have quick fixes, no matter what you hear on late-night infomercials. Heart disease, diabetes, cancer, depression, etc., do not just come out of nowhere, although they can feel like they do. Conducting research on which interventions are most effective to treat these diseases becomes quite difficult and costly. Researchers track patients for many years, without making them feel like they are being stalked, and such tracking typically takes an extraordinary amount of resources that should be used wisely.

Apparently Finnish scientists did not get that memo.

A recently published long-term Finnish study demonstrated that young bullies later possess greater antisocial (in the sense of antisocietal and aggressive) tendencies. Don't get us wrong; we fully support research and resources being devoted to the issue of bullying. The problem with the Finnish study is that finding that bullies demonstrate greater antisocial tendencies is like finding that men have a greater tendency to watch action movies, women have a greater tendency to watch romantic comedies, and no one has a tendency to watch Katherine Heigl movies.

Fortunately, this study had some interesting findings, the most notable being that not only is bullying associated with antisocial behaviors, bullying can actually *cause* these behaviors, by making bullies more aggressive than they already were. In other words, preventing bullies from bullying can actually help the bullies, just as preventing alcoholics from drinking can help them appear to be less fun at parties.

Between research demonstrating the long-term effects of bullying on others and well-known cases of children dying by suicide because of being bullied, there has been a crackdown on bullies. As with most activities that get cracked down on, technology has been embraced as a tool to subvert the crackdown. Some have asked whether resources would be better devoted to understanding and treating the cause of bullying rather than merely punishing it.

Although punitive measures have, after all, completely eliminated the drug problem, right?

37

Why Didn't They Call It Uranus?

Of the few names that can be used to describe an element, a God, *and* a planet (we'll let you fellow geeks figure out all four of these terms), none has caused the pervasive harm throughout history that mercury has, despite centuries of society and physicians thinking that a spoonful of mercury helped the medicine go down. Its list of famous victims would make *People* magazine jealous. From King Charles II and George III to composers like Beethoven and Mozart to great leaders like Abraham Lincoln and Napoleon Bonaparte and even scientists Isaac Newton and Michael Faraday, mercury's reach has known no bounds in place or time—kind of like a Barry Manilow song. Despite thousands of years of progress and many medical recommendations regarding mercury exposure and consumption, just a few years ago actor Jeremy Piven—yes, we don't remember him, either—had to leave a Broadway show owing to mercury poisoning from excess sushi consumption. So maybe sticking with California rolls isn't such a bad idea.

Mercury is primarily obtained from cinnabar, which we were disappointed to find out did not contain delicious icing and a month's supply of shame. Mercury's main use throughout the eighteenth and nineteenth centuries was in the hatting industry. Exposure to mercury ultimately caused tremors and mental illness in hatmakers. In fact, the term "mad as a hatter" served as inspiration for Lewis

Carroll. Interestingly enough, the Mad Hatter was portrayed by Johnny Depp, who was expected by some to play Queen frontman Freddie *Mercury*—and the circle is complete.

As if mercury's omnipresence in mining, sea life, and numerous products hasn't been bad enough, physicians are guilty of adding to the problem. Go figure that cheap, mercury-filled thermometers occasionally leak or break. So if you weren't sick *before* your temperature was checked . . .

Recently some parents have feared that the minute amounts of mercury contained in vaccines are potentially dangerous. While there's no evidence that the minuscule amount of mercury in vaccines is harmful, and the research clearly shows that the benefits of vaccines are substantial, the debate continues as to whether mercury use should be limited in vaccines. The expert opinions on this are constantly changing, making the whole debate rather . . . mercurial.

See what we did there?

38

Kill Your Television . . . Except If Watching *Modern Family*

We have come to expect that certain behaviors link with certain outcomes, leading to recommendations around all these behaviors. Smoking increases cancer. Lack of exercise increases obesity. Watching Fox News increases ignorance. We have enjoyed observing these trends as much as we enjoy a good Netflix binge. So boy were we bummed when we came across a study that demonstrated that increased television viewing is associated with depression. Fortunately we were able to drown these feelings by streaming back-to-back episodes of *Lost*.

What would have been more interesting is if this study had distinguished association and causation. In other words, we know that increased television viewing is associated with depression, which we can't solely blame on *Two and a Half Men*. Is this because watching television a lot makes people depressed, or because those who are depressed watch television a lot? Or could it be that watching lots of television can make people depressed, and depressed people then watch television more? Which came first? We tried asking a chicken, which referred the question to its predecessor.

Increased television viewing has actually been associated with far more than depression. Heavy amounts of television watching have been associated with obesity and even premature death. One of the authors of this book even published an article in *The New York Times* examining whether depiction of violence in media, including on television, increases violence in children.

Now consider this: If a medication were found to increase obesity, early death, violence, and depression, it would be expeditiously pulled off the market—after a few years, since the drug company needs to make some money off it first, of course. But, much like Charlton Heston and his guns, most Americans will give you their remote controls when you pry them from their cold, dead hands.

Back to television's impact on the brain . . . watching television has been shown to cause changes in brain waves potentially associated with depression. Such changes are not seen with more engaging types of entertainment, like reading a book, playing a sport, or having sex. While watching TV in moderation is fine, try to avoid watching the four hours of TV per day that most Americans do after work. Instead, crack open a novel, go to the basketball court, or get a little freaky in the bedroom. Just remember, if you choose to videotape the latter (à la Kim Kardashian), don't take too long or you might just end up sitting in front of the TV again later.

39

Holy Mackerel!

In our practice and research we have come across hundreds of examples of "natural" cures peddled by charlatans looking to make a buck. Most of these fad cures do not last longer than the length of their infomercials. Typically, enough people have a lack of success that the fad dies—or the people that try it do. Rarely do we come across a supposed cure that lives on, especially when the cure is alive itself.

Every year in India tens of thousands gather for the privilege of swallowing raw fish, and we're not talking sushi here. More specifically, a family in India has claimed to have a cure for asthma. The treatment is pretty simple; all you have to do is come to Hyderabad, a city in southern India, on a specific day, determined by astrologers, and swallow a five-to-eight-centimeter live fish that has been stuffed with a secret herbal paste mixed with blessed well water (none of that bottled swill). Then you take the secret mix home and consume it as part of a special, restrictive diet for forty-five days. Oh, and then you have to do this all over again every year for three years. BOOM, cured.

You would think that jumping through all these hoops would require some evidence, especially since this treatment, if followed "properly," supposedly has a 100 percent cure rate for asthma. If this process doesn't cure you, that means that *you* must have done something wrong. Perhaps the extraordinary growth in attendance is due to the most surprising fact about this treatment: The family that administers it does not charge a cent. It turns out this cure is rooted in religious enlightenment. In the nineteenth century, a holy man revealed his religious insights into the fish swallowing, and its popularity has been growing ever since.

The government of India actually sponsors shuttles to the fish-swallowing ceremony. Despite lack of evidence supporting this treatment, no one has documented that it is harmful, either. Truly, faith in the treatment can have a powerful effect in itself.

So maybe Dr. Seuss shouldn't have been so criticized for his first draft: "One fish, two fish, swallow fish, cure asthma."

40

Take the Lead.
It's Prescription.

These days, most people know about lead poisoning. Actually, that knowledge is not new. In fact, ancient Romans were aware of lead poisoning and tried to minimize their slaves' exposure to lead. Despite this awareness, some experts theorize that lead exposure brought down the whole empire—and here we always thought it was repeated waves of German marauders. In fact, it has been suggested that lead caused the great Julius Caesar to be not so great in the bedroom. Despite his choice of concubines he produced only one offspring, Caesar Augustus. Given what we know about that offspring, perhaps it's good that he was an only child. Caesar Augustus himself was sterile, ending possibly the most powerful family line in history, other than the Bushes.

The awareness of lead poisoning did not keep millions from being poisoned over the years. Lead is an extremely useful metal. What's a little anemia, diffuse pain, and psychosis for the sake of having a nice paint job, right? Although we sympathize with the mistakes of ancient civilizations, as their knowledge was limited, it is hard to have a Bronze Age without the bronze. What we take greater issue with is not only lead's more recent presence in all sorts of household materials, but its presence in many medicines themselves. At least now FDA-regulated prescriptions are lead-free, but many nonregulated medications might still be contaminated. It goes without saying that we're not big fans of curing the disease by killing the patient. (And not only because the paperwork is so laborious.)

As you might expect, business ambitions overcame health and environmental ethics. In the 1920s, despite more than two thousand years of knowledge regarding the dangers of lead and health experts warning about those dangers, potent liquid lead was incorporated into gasoline—surely the only time when a need for fuel has harmed the planet. Only after fifty years of research could health and environmental experts overcome the energy lobby, and these changes in the law immediately prompted the production of cleaner-burning engines. Somehow industry and the economy went on, despite energy companies arguing that they wouldn't. We're sure that after two thousand years the lesson has finally been learned—although this doesn't do Caesar any good.

41

You Won't Always Be Able to Control Everything

We often see people who want to know the gender of the child before the delivery; it's hard to invest in a lot of pink or blue stuff without a liberal return policy. Some, however, have decided to take it a step further and try to regulate the sex of the child before conception. While we appreciate the effort, as fathers we have given up trying to control every aspect of our children's lives, as they took control of us the day they were born.

Gender selection, otherwise known as "family balancing" so it doesn't sound as bad as the methods some parents in certain Asian countries employ, has been around as long as there have been children—although the techniques have progressed from the whole "send the child in a basket down the river to be found and adopted by royalty and eventually lead a revolution" thing.

The techniques range from "natural" to highly technical. (We put "natural" in quotes because "natural gender selection" sounds like being "a little pregnant.") To have a boy—which, per our parents, is definitely not the preferred option—eat a more alkaline diet full of sodium and potassium. For a girl, eat a more acidic diet high in magnesium, and of course, sugar and spice and everything nice. Another technique involves timing of sex based on the ovulatory cycle. Sperm with male genes are faster, but more fragile—go figure—while female sperm are built to last. Supposedly, if sex is timed so there is some delay between bumping uglies and ovulation, tougher female sperm have a better chance of outlasting the male sperm, similar to how our wives outlast us in any argument we have ever had.

Another technique we came across involves the timing of doin' it based on the Chinese—surprise, surprise—calendar. Techniques now have advanced to taking a bunch of hormonal drugs, having eggs harvested, fertilizing embryos outside the body, and selecting those of a specific gender. As pleasant as all that sounds, as parents we have learned how much unpredictability there is with children. We have also learned the value in loving them for just who they are, regardless of gender, personality, or their absolute disregard for their parents' repeated requests to wipe their feet before they come inside. But for those who feel they want only a child of a certain gender and are not willing to adopt, feel free to implement any or all of the above techniques. Or, simply just enjoy the process of baby making.

42

What If They Were Lactating?

When we first read this study we were envious. While our research projects in college and medical school involved test tubes and MRI machines, the authors of this study closely studied the abilities of lap dancers. More specifically, they probed into whether strippers earned greater tips depending on whether they were ovulating. What made the authors grope for an answer to this question was the fact that one of the authors worked at a strip club and noticed that the strippers to whom he had to give tampons tended to earn fewer tips. Since he was also a student in evolutionary psychology—unlike the strippers, who were all putting themselves through law school—he decided to research this more formally. After all, he needed to use his research-grant money somehow, and they say to do what you love.

Many could make fun of this research topic: from resources spent on studying such an esoteric topic, to someone receiving lap dances and calling it scientific. In this case, however, we can defend the seemingly indefensible. First of all, the study wasn't performed in the way many readers might think/want/fantasize. Surveys of strippers were performed to learn about their tips and ovulatory cycles, so at least there were some formal parameters beyond measuring grinds and thrusts. Amazingly, strippers who were ovulating made approximately $30 more per hour in tips than strippers who were menstruating, and not just because the latter kept their bottoms on.

This finding actually has major implications. For most of intelligent man's (oxymoron?) history, it was felt that human beings were the one species that did not give overt signs that they were "in heat." This study suggests otherwise: There is some form of nonverbal communication, possibly an unknown pheromone, or the strippers' breasts are more engorged. Alternatively, during peak production times strippers might just be more lax on the "no hands" policy!

Typically when any scientific study is performed, whatever question is answered is followed by the next question that should be investigated. In this case, it is identifying how women demonstrate they are in heat. We don't think they will have trouble finding male volunteers.

43

Well, Who Is Going to Open the Pickle Jar?

Without knowing it, we learn to accept certain basic tenets in life. The sun will rise tomorrow, Twinkies will last forever, and fifteen minutes can save you 15 percent on car insurance. Another of life's fundamentals is that a child is produced by a man and a woman. To be clear, we are not commenting on the definition of marriage or the proper structure of a nuclear family—especially as two of the authors live in San Francisco and recognize that atypical families are the new typical.

As physicians, we are just saying that biologically, even with in vitro fertilization, producing a child has always required the genetic material of a man, a woman, and Barry White songs. This has made some wonder: Is there a way to get rid of the man (and therefore bring up the average intelligence of the child)? Apparently some scientists have figured out how to incorporate genetic material from either gender into a mouse egg to create a mouse embryo, and are currently working to impregnate mice with those embryos. Which is brave, because it ain't easy being a single-mouse household (mousehold?) these days.

While we are avid supporters of female empowerment, we do get a little nervous about technology that makes men no longer necessary to perpetuate the species and requires us to justify our existence. In the end, we know that women will need men; what would we all do without football, beer, and war? Besides, the old saying isn't nearly as catchy if it's changed to "Men, can't live with them . . . and that's why we're developing a novel approach for incorporating genetic material from another woman into a female egg."

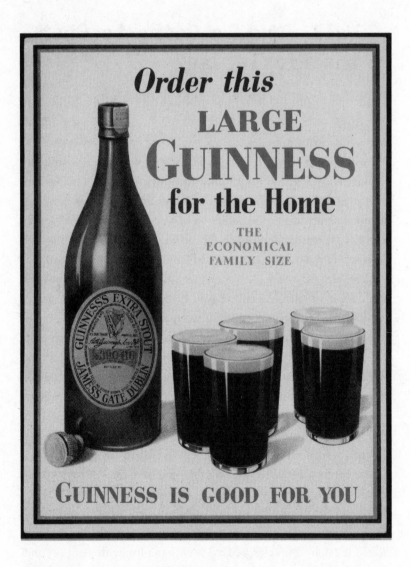

Advertisement for Guinness, extoling its health benefits.
Credit: Wellcome Library, London. Obtained from: Creative Commons by 4.0.

44

Don't Blame the Irish

We always found it interesting that doctors used to recommend clearly harmful substances to patients. However, this practice reaches a whole new level when the harmful advice is given to pregnant women; you are poisoning for two, after all. In the 1920s, back in (not so) Great Britain, physicians used to recommend Guinness to pregnant women, and not just the hormonal ones who needed to calm down. We realize that in Europe they tend to start drinking alcohol earlier, but before they turn zero might be going too far.

The belief was that Guinness's high level of iron could help support blood-cell production in pregnant women, thereby making it healthy, just as consuming fast-food hamburgers is good for you because of the vitamin C in the ketchup. Physicians made the same recommendations to those donating blood. While Guinness is more desirable than juice and cookies, we question the wisdom in recommending beer to those who have just given up a pint of blood, as it may make them more unsteady or drunk-dial their ex.

The ironic aspect of this recommendation is that Guinness does not have very much iron at all. The typical pint contains 0.3 milligrams, which is approximately 3 percent of the U.S. recommended daily allowance. In other words, to get even the recommended daily intake of iron for a nonpregnant person, it would take about thirty pints of Guinness . . . as if pregnant women didn't have to pee enough already.

Interestingly, Guinness lager has been demonstrated to have health benefits over stout, at least in dogs with heart disease—we won't even get into how we found this study. Researchers believe the benefit is due to the higher level of antioxidants in Guinness lager, but physicians will not go so far as to again make health claims. Fool me once, shame on you; fool me twice, I was probably drunk.

45

And It Makes You Look Cool

If you are not smart enough to realize that smoking is bad for your health, at least you may not get too much stupider. For years, numerous studies actually showed a benefit to smoking, that it decreases future risk of dementia—and not just because most smokers don't live long enough to get dementia. First, we wonder why this was even studied; it's not as if showing a possible benefit, such as reducing the risk of dementia, will suddenly kick us back to the *Mad Men* age of doctor-encouraged smoking. Plus, we think it's unlikely that smokers regularly review medical literature, considering that they can't even pay attention to the large warning on the pack. For that rare brilliant smoker—the president of the United States and former editor of the *Harvard Law Review* Barack Obama has been known to take the occasional puff—any theoretical benefit is nothing weighed against all the cancers, cardiovascular disease, and, worst of all, yellow teeth.

In the last few years, though, the literature has seemed to show an *increased* risk of dementia in those who smoke. Why the difference? It might have to do with the fact that most of the studies showing the benefit were affiliated with tobacco companies and that most showing harm were not. But it's not like a tobacco company would ever do anything immoral just to support their business. That's just crazy talk.

There may be other ways to reconcile this conflict (of interest).

While smoking is more likely harmful to the brain because it can clog blood vessels, nicotine has been shown to help reduce cognitive decline in dementia patients. But then there's the pesky side effect that nicotine can elevate blood pressure and heart rate, and, of course, it remains very addictive. Fortunately, marijuana has been demonstrated to have the same dementia-reducing benefits without being as addictive ... or so we've been told. Perhaps the biggest benefit of this is that no one has to say they have glaucoma to get a prescription for medicinal marijuana; they can just say they do not want to get dementia forty years from now. Though it may be hard to convince anyone that you should be allowed to smoke weed because it can make you smarter. Or maybe not. Who knows, maybe the maker of Doritos will sponsor that next study.

46

Not Just Good for
Serving Revenge

Most of the supposed cures we investigate are medicinal, but when all those treatments are exhausted, one might feel left in the cold. At least that gives one more cure to try. In fact, cryotherapy, or cold therapy, has been demonstrated to have some pretty cool uses, although some suggested uses of cold therapy might make our male readers' genitalia shrivel.

The mechanism behind most uses of cryotherapy is that making cells colder slows or stops the cellular metabolism, which can reduce harmful inflammation, or, if cold enough, can even cause cell death. In addition, by hardening the areas that are frozen, cryotherapy can help remove lesions. Overall, cryotherapy has been demonstrated to help with muscular strains, cancer, and herpes. But before you shove some ice down your pants and fire up your Tinder app, you should know that cryotherapy doesn't get rid of herpes; it only helps with the removal of various types of warts. Recent studies demonstrate that cryotherapy may be even more effective for plantar (foot) warts and a little cheaper and easier to get than the traditional treatment of liquid nitrogen. Now, before you go all MacGyver on your warts, you should know that it can take a couple of months . . . so maybe just get that pedicure before you date the guy with the foot fetish.

What gives us shivers is some of the other suggested "treatments" based on cryotherapy, including cryogenics, or the study of effects of very low temperatures. In addition to "cryogenics" sounding like it comes from L. Ron Hubbard, so do some of its uses. Many have investigated cryogenics as a tool for immortality, allowing us to preserve those who undergo the freezing procedure. Supposedly Walt Disney is to remain in stasis until the appropriate time for re*animation*. While there is a fistful of irony in Walt Disney wanting to become animated, we'd be more impressed if, upon revival, he requested a private screening of *Frozen*.

47

Does the Carpet Match the Drapes?

As a society, we obsess about so many aspects of our looks that it's no surprise that some people start to feel gloomy at the thought of going gray. While some women learn to accept "the change" and some men learn to accept that they are now more attractive to women who have "daddy issues," others feel compelled to dye their hair to hide their colorful secret. Then, there are a few for whom dyeing is almost as bad as dying, and so they strive for another way to shed the gray.

Fixing gray hair is not so black-and-white, though, as there can be many different causes of the graying, and not all have to do with being a member of the Republican Party. While all gray hair is from loss of activity in melanocytes, the same cells in our skin that cause tanning, the reason they lose this activity varies as much as hairstyles. Possible reasons can include: vitamin B_{12} deficiency (vegans beware!), which can cause anemia; abnormal thyroid function that you can also blame for making you fat; and a high level of stress, which has been labeled as a possible cause of pretty much any health problem ever.

The many different causes don't stop snake oil, or perhaps in this case hair oil, salesmen from pushing their various cures. Supposed remedies for gray hair include colloid copper and blackstrap molasses, for those of you who feel like consuming metal and other strange substances. Topical "cures" include an onion-and-lemon-juice mixture applied to the head, for those of you who want to completely repel women (or make hummus).

Perhaps those with gray hair would more appreciate what they have if they just looked at someone who is bald. It's like the old adage "Once I cried, for I had no shoes. Then I met a man who had no feet—so I took his shoes."

48

We Are Not Suggesting You Suck on It

Many substances have been found to suppress cancer cells, but few are as interesting as this one. A substance in breast milk, known as human alpha-lactalbumin or HAMLET, has been found to have potent anticancer activity, without the sedative effects of the Shakespeare play. This makes HAMLET the only anticancer chemical produced naturally by humans. This also makes it the anticancer chemical that is most fun to pronounce.

For many years it has been known that children who are breast-fed have a lower incidence of cancer. One reason for this might be that antibodies found in breast milk can boost the immune system, which can help suppress cancer cells. With the discovery of HAMLET and its tumor-fighting ability, there may be implications beyond the development of babies' immune systems. For example, studies have suggested that HAMLET can possibly shrink tumors and prolong life in cases of brain and bladder cancer. To confirm these findings more studies will have to be done, which may require greater production of breast milk. We anticipate no lack of male volunteers to assist in that study.

One fact that makes us skeptical of the potential of HAMLET in cancer treatment is that hundreds of chemicals have been found to suppress tumors, ranging from capsaicin—the spicy component of peppers—to marijuana, which has been shown to cure everything.

None of these treatments have yet reached prime time as a primary cancer treatment, though. Conspiracy theorists suggest that this is because there is not as much profit to be made by marketing widely available, naturally occurring chemicals. Should those conspiracy theorists get cancer, instead of chemotherapy, surgery, and radiation, they are welcome to try breast milk, hot peppers, and marijuana instead. We would rather pay a little extra, and just enjoy those other chemicals on the side, although maybe not all at the same time.

49

So That's What the
Track Marks Are From

Dealing with chronic pain and want some relief? Are prescription pills no longer doing it for you? The solution is easy: Simply turn to needles!

The practice of acupuncture has been passed down for thousands of years. While it originated in Eastern cultures, it has become more commonly accepted and even standardized in modern medicine teaching programs, although that doesn't stop the occasional amateur from trying. If an acupuncturist is working out of a car, and because of the low overhead is able to charge you a discount, be ready to get what you paid for. Don't be surprised when the acupuncturist asks you to share needles as part of a cost-savings program.

Ancient acupuncture was based on the notion that we have imbalances in qi, which in addition to being the basic life force is also one of the best words you can play in Scrabble. This imbalance was likely the original "chemical imbalance." Rather than the imbalance being corrected with medications, the idea was that needles would redirect the energy. The current theory behind acupuncture is that the needles stimulate nerves, which can release neurotransmitters, endorphins, etc. And of course the whole practice is based on the belief that there are no negative consequences of sticking needles in nerve centers.

Like many "alternative" therapies, acupuncture has been suggested to help pain, nausea, depression, infertility, cancer, stroke, etc. Unlike many other therapies, though, acupuncture actually has a bit of evidence behind it. In fact, acupuncture has become so accepted that the term "alternative medicine" has fallen out of favor to describe it. For a while "complementary medicine" was in vogue, but for some reason that wasn't enough, so eventually everyone settled on "integrative medicine."

Whoever is doing this labeling seems to be expending quite a lot of effort.

50

Good for the Birds, Bad for the Worms

It's the age-old question: Should you finish that assignment or finish the new season of *Orange Is the New Black*? While the answer to what is the *right* thing to do still may elude us, we do have some insight into the effects of procrastination. According to a recent study, those who turned in assignments earlier actually got better grades. Apparently schoolteachers don't grade like Olympic judges, saving the best scores until the end. Then there's of course the Russian judge who cared less about who went first than who bribed the French judge first.

We had to wonder who would spend money to perform such a study and were surprised to learn that it was the typically financially conservative United Kingdom. Spending money on studies like this would be as wasteful as spending large amounts of tax money to fund an outdated royalty that has no current relevance in modern politics. Wait a minute. . . .

The source of funding was even more interesting in that it was actually funded by a business school in the UK. Full disclosure: One of your physician authors went to business school—yes, he's a grad-school addict—and it was once discussed in class how some business schools occasionally feel insecure regarding the level of their standards compared with their legal or medical school brethren. Performing "studies" of this kind does not help their cause and only teaches business school students—the future citizens of Wall Street—to spend other people's money in frivolous and risky ways. Wait another minute. . . .

So when your junior-high-school kids don't want to do their homework right after school and try to put it off until late at night, just show them this "scientific" study demonstrating that they might get worse grades because of the delay. Hopefully this will change their minds . . . but make sure you don't procrastinate doing it. In addition, the same author who went to business school is an emergency-room doctor, and it's clear that in the ER procrastination can have some trivial consequences, such as death. We were tempted to perform a similar study in the ER to more dramatically show the effects of procrastination, but we couldn't get anyone to sign up on time.

51

You Mean It Won't Fall Off?

While there are many legends about the health risks of masturbation, few people seem to discuss all the benefits, beyond the obvious immediate one. Generally, masturbation is regarded as a vice or a sin, perhaps out of fear that if it was thought to be beneficial, and a TV was installed across from the toilet, a vast majority of men would have no reason to ever leave the bathroom.

Masturbating is a double-edged sword, with various risks and benefits. Like many practices, the more you do yourself the ultimate favor, the fewer the benefits and the greater the risks—and not just carpal tunnel. Some studies show that those who masturbate have lower testosterone levels than either those who do not masturbate or those who engage in intercourse. And we know from other research that lower testosterone is actually associated with a decrease in sex drive. In the other hand, whoops, we mean *on* the other hand: Some data suggest that masturbation can help prime people for sex, although most men really need no priming.

Another possible benefit of masturbation is the lowering of cortisol, the main stress hormone, which can help regulate blood sugar, cholesterol, fat storage, and blood pressure, all of which can benefit the heart. Knowing this could certainly change how you deal with the next stressful work situation, for better or for awkward. The good news is that these cardiovascular benefits of masturbation also confirm the theorized association between a man's heart and his penis.

Higher frequency of masturbation has also been associated with lower levels of prostate cancer, presumably due to stored semen not languishing near the prostate for so long that it builds up "pollutants." Masturbation is therefore nature's Drano, with both often ending up as deposits in the toilet.

The last advantage of gettin' it on with yourself is the flexibility as to where and when it can be performed, not needing to be timed with another person, or, if you are really lucky, several other people. With all this opportunity, the key to preserving the benefits of anything so amply available is to practice everything in moderation— even moderation itself. So if you do have the problem of masturbating excessively, at least remember to take an occasional bathroom break, or in this case, a break from the bathroom.

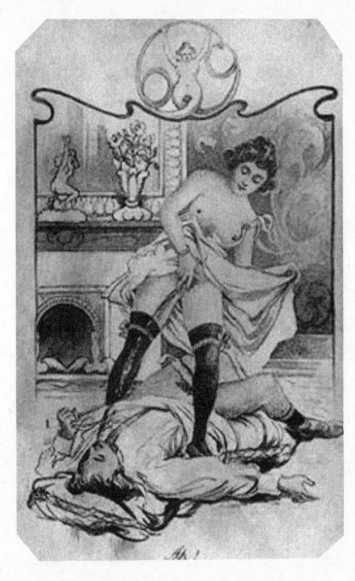

One way to drink urine. Originally from:
upload.wikimedia.org/wikipedia/commons/f/fd/Pissing-illustration.jpg. Public Domain.

52

How Many Licks Does It Take?

Before there were simple laboratory tests that incorporated bodily fluids, the easiest way to check for certain abnormalities was to use one's senses of smell and taste. Increased iron in the blood could make blood taste metallic. Increased sugar in blood or urine could taste sweet or smell like alcohol. Cyanide poisoning can smell like bitter almonds (but please don't try the taste test at home in this case). In fact, bitter almonds are actually illegal in the United States because they really do contain a small amount of cyanide. When we were taught in medical school this pearl about cyanide smelling like bitter almonds, we could not help but wonder how they expected us to recognize the smell of something not available in the United States. But we quickly got used to unreasonable expectations, as we were also expected to work one hundred hours a week and not get bitter ourselves.

In general, we are not fans of anything that requires tasting bodily fluids to make the diagnosis. Something about that conflicts with our ingrained notions of sterility and contact precautions, or, just to be frank, it's simply disgusting. Even the thought of having to taste fluids is enough to make us upchuck the boogie. Equally nauseating would be licking sweat to see if it tastes salty. There was a time when even that practice was on the table—meaning the practice of licking, not the salt.

Sweat is typically comprised of fluids and electrolytes, namely sodium and chloride, which are the key ingredients in salt. Adjusting the amount of these salts can vary the taste significantly, as we have learned from every night we cooked in medical school.

Cystic fibrosis is a severe disease that causes secretions from many organs, like the lungs and pancreas, to become thick and plug ducts. This defect results in an excess amount of chloride on the skin, which is the least of the problems in cystic fibrosis. In the past, doctors would taste sweat to diagnose cystic fibrosis at a very early age in patients, when the disease could be mollified through treatment. As there are more sophisticated techniques for measuring the exact amount of chloride in sweat these days, fortunately we no longer have to rely on the sophistication of a physician's palate.

The first "improvement" on this tasting technique was to place a patient in a chamber in which the temperature and humidity were raised until the patient was tortured enough to induce sweat—in this case actually forcing the patient to take a licking.

53

Try Not to Bruise It

Even Duran Duran knows what a reflex is. The most widely recognized reflex involves tapping a reflex hammer just under the knee, causing the leg to kick out, and not just as revenge for being hit with a hammer. There are many more reflexes, though, ranging from gastrointestinal, such as having to go number two after a meal, to respiratory, such as breathing automatically. Reflexes can be as unusual as your eyelids closing spontaneously when you sneeze (and it's not because the eyes will pop out if they are open) to the sensual loss of muscle control in an orgasm. Perhaps the leg kicking out isn't the most widely recognized reflex after all. . . .

The basic concept of the reflex is that a nerve gets stimulated—or in the case of the orgasm, something else gets repeatedly stimulated—and a signal is transmitted in the body. Those who practice reflexology massage believe that by stimulating certain areas they can control other areas of the body. Now, whether the reflexology masseuse will stimulate the orgasm-inducing areas depends on the masseur and whether she also believes in the practice of happy endings . . . not to mention how much the massage is costing.

Specifically, reflexologists believe that through the application of pressure to certain areas of the hands and feet, all other parts of the body can be relaxed. Perhaps there is some truth there, as who doesn't like a foot massage? Even the reflexologists seem to enjoy touching their clients' sweaty, smelly, often fungal-infested feet, or maybe they just enjoy that they can charge a higher hourly rate than a nurse. Although reflexology is rooted in thousands of years of Chinese tradition and is not just an effort to get health-insurance companies to reimburse for foot massages, current research does not show a specific therapeutic result other than just feeling good. As we have learned, though, if you just want to feel good, there are some *far* better reflexes.

54

The Only Time You Would
Rather Deal with a Prick

How sweet it is! Literally.

Diabetes, or "the sugar," as referred to by our great-grandparents, is a disorder of excessively high amounts of glucose, the body's main form of sugar, in the blood. Having persistently high blood sugar contributes to kidney failure, vision loss, Wilford Brimley infomercials, heart disease, and many other health problems. Who would have thought a lifetime of soda and ice cream could eventually cause health issues?

There are actually two forms of diabetes. Type I diabetes, formerly known as juvenile diabetes, predominantly occurs in youth. In this type of diabetes, antibodies destroy the cells in the pancreas that are responsible for insulin production. Insulin is a hormone that reduces blood sugar by either storing the sugar in tissues or allowing cells to use the sugar as energy. When the insulin-producing cells are destroyed, blood sugar becomes progressively elevated and can reach extremely high levels. Since the cells are not able to use sugar, they use fat as energy, which creates acid as a by-product. Type I diabetics are therefore usually skinny and hungry, and their blood is full of acid . . . and not the kind of acid one can get high off (unless you count their extreme sugar high).

Type II diabetes, formerly known as adult-onset diabetes, occurs when the body still makes insulin, but becomes progressively resistant to it. There are multiple mechanisms for this, but basically there is increased insulin resistance when there is excess body fat. Sadly, this is no longer known as adult-onset diabetes owing to the prevalence of childhood obesity, causing an increasing amount of Type II diabetes in children—as if overweight kids didn't already have it hard enough. Some have proposed calling Alzheimer's disease Type III diabetes, because it relates to an insulin resistance in the brain. Personally, we're not a fan of making a third just because the first two are so successful. We're lookin' at you, *The Hangover* guys.

In diabetics, the high amounts of sugar overwhelm the kidney and cause sugar to leak into the urine. While testing blood sugar these days is easy—a mere finger prick—there was a time when performing a blood test was more complicated. As a simpler alternative, referred to in the "How Many Licks Does It Take?" chapter, physicians used to check for high blood sugar by looking for it in the urine, or to be accurate, *tasting* it in the urine. And you thought being a physician was all glamour.

Despite how disgusting this sounds, if it meant diabetes could be diagnosed and treated, it was worth it to save lives. Tastes great, less . . . killing?

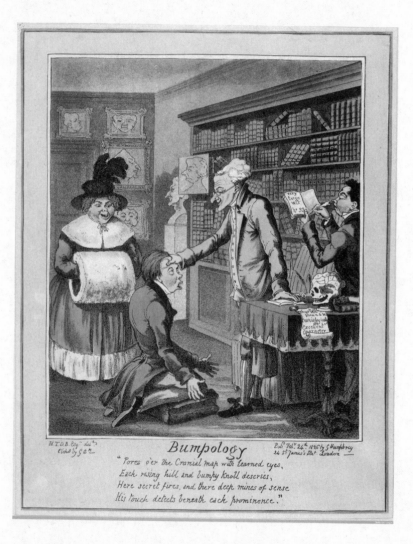

Phrenology, how the shape of the skull affects personality, in practice.
Credit: Wellcome Library, London. Obtained from: Creative Commons by 4.0.

55

It's All in Your Head

Don't you hate when people ogle your shape? It just makes you want to say, "Hey, there's a brain here!" But what do you say when the shape they are obsessed with *is* the shape of your brain?

Turns out there is an entire "science" obsessed with the shape of the brain, or more specifically, its container, the skull. The science is in quotes because it is more accurately described as a "pseudoscience," which technically is defined as something that is presented as scientific, without that little thing called "evidence" behind it. Other famous pseudosciences include astrology, palm reading, and pretty much anything promoted by Jenny McCarthy.

The first thing to do when establishing a pseudoscience is to give it an official-sounding name. For example, while we were in residency, we closely studied "megatranquilology," or the study of how to relax, any chance we had. The study of how the shape of the skull affects personality is known as phrenology, which apparently is not just the title of a Roots album. Phrenology became popular in the nineteenth century, and is about as useful as its contemporaries cholera and typhoid.

The next step is to use a pseudoscience to try and take advantage of others. In early phrenology, it was argued that the shape of certain ethnic group's—specifically Europeans'—skulls determined that they were more evolved. A German—there it is again!—physician originally founded phrenology. We've heard of another German who promoted similar beliefs a hundred years later.

Fortunately, often some good has come from pseudosciences. Phrenology was one of the original studies of personality and helped lead to evidence-based psychology and psychiatry. The study of psychiatry has helped millions—in addition to helping two of the authors find ways to help patients without actually feeling their patients' skulls.

56

Forget the Eye of the Tiger

Charlie Sheen famously proclaimed to have tiger blood running through his veins. He was also famous for certain other activities outside of his acting. Tiger Woods was famous for similar activities outside of his main profession as well. Coincidence? Or is there something about tigers that make the women say, "They're g-r-r-r-e-a-t!"

Apparently, for hundreds of years tiger penis has been considered an aphrodisiac, and its consumption is believed to improve sexual prowess. Of course, we discovered this only when researching this book. We also learned that this belief is more common in Asian countries. Insert ethnically insensitive and offensive penis joke here.

Tiger penis, in addition to bull penis and turtle penis—we have to wonder if the latter is slower to work but may be harder overall—are still served as cuisine in some countries. Preparation involves slicing up a penis and putting it in soup, as wives often threaten to do. Some diners have been known to spend thousands of dollars for a gourmet dish, which is surprising considering how many Internet pop-up ads say they can do the same to your penis for far less.

Despite this expensive demand, consuming tiger penis is condemned by most societies, as it contributes to poaching. While we fully support this condemnation, is poaching really the main reason we should not eat penis? And what about poached penis?

The most unusual recipe we found involves using not only the penis but also the testicles, letting them soak for weeks in wine, and sipping small amounts of the wine nightly. All we can say is that to drink this, it sure takes a lot of balls.

57

They Eventually Get
Their Revenge

We have always been amazed at how some researchers feel compelled to research the trivial or the obvious. So when we found a study showing that science "nerds" are more likely to be virgins, we hit the jackpot. Plus, having been science nerds ourselves, we felt that this hit close to home. If only there were some science nerds whom women found attractive. Wait, we call those doctors and computer programmers.

This does not mean that a science nerd can't get any "action," or that there aren't non-nerds who are compelled to abstain from sex. The point is that if you are smart and into science, you have a couple of strikes against you. We certainly learned nothing new from this research, as we can remember countless nights when we were studying or at the research lab while our friends were at parties or clubs. Here we were wasting our time learning how to save lives.

Apparently, this ability to "delay gratification" is actually an asset. A Stanford study demonstrated that over the course of forty years, those who as children were best able to delay gratification—by not eating a marshmallow so they can have two later—were more successful as adults. The delayers had higher SAT scores, lower levels of substance abuse, less obesity, better response to stress, better social skills, and were overall happier. For everything there is balance, though, and even Warren Buffett—one of the richest men in the world, who is known for his patience—recognizes the pointlessness in "saving up sex for old age."

So if you are a science nerd, and worry about your prospects, perhaps you can improve your odds by surrounding yourself with those more likely to have sex. Fortunately, the study also showed who was having the most rolls in the hay—female art students—though some of them may come with their own set of issues. If that doesn't bother you, consider taking an acting class . . . if you can handle the drama.

58

You Don't Need to
Re-prove Gravity

We have nothing against adrenaline junkies. We do have something against spending time and money in research proving that obviously dangerous practices are indeed dangerous. We found multiple research studies demonstrating dangers of bungee jumping and skydiving. Apparently, individuals who engage in these activities suffer eye, head, and neck injuries, and even death. Thank goodness these findings have been recorded and can dissuade future potential participants, who we are sure do their research and logically consider all these consequences.

So why do people do these extreme sports? Activities that are life-threatening cause a release of certain neurotransmitters, like epinephrine and norepinephrine, which stimulate receptors to cause many changes in physiology. The heart beats faster, blood flow to many tissues increases, and because of the neurotransmitters' similarity to dopamine, even the brain's pleasure center gets stimulated—hence the desire for the repeated stimulation. Certain illicit drugs, like cocaine and amphetamines, have similar effects. Needless to say, we do not endorse drug use because of drugs' effects on the body and brain. Bungee jumping and skydiving can have bad effects on the body and brain as well, though those effects tend to be a little more sudden.

If those neurotransmitters are pleasurable, why do we not all seek these activities? Because we are all different, duh! It's the same reason we do not all become drug addicts. The type of stimulation we receive can vary. For example, we do not find performing research that reaffirms the dangers of bungee jumping and skydiving very stimulating, but clearly someone does. While we do not have a lot of appreciation for research that does not have nearly as much impact on society as its subjects' impact on pavement, we will stop short of suggesting that such researchers should go take a leap. Because we know if they do, someone else will feel a need to study it.

59

Are They Crooked?

Your spinal cord controls all the movements of your body. It is a tiny, fragile piece of soft tissue nestled in between hard jagged bones, from which nerves radiate everywhere in your body. If the spinal cord or these nerves are damaged, paralysis or even death can occur. So why would people voluntarily subject themselves to getting these bones manipulated in various directions, and pay handsomely for the privilege? Are they being manipulated themselves?

Though it is commonly believed that physicians look down on chiropractors and refer to them as "medical-school rejects," modern Western medicine has actually come a long way in recent decades and is more open to chiropractic medicine. Still, spinal issues have remained a huge pain in the neck for many physicians, with therapies being limited to addictive pain medicines and risky surgery, both of which often lead to recidivism. While return visits may make a physician more money, it's bad for patients and the health care system, so we'll take any solution to help straighten out this mess—and patients' spines.

Chiropractic medicine, like many health professions, goes wrong when it purports to cure more than evidence suggests, such as high blood pressure, menstrual cramps, asthma, acne, and ear infections. The theory is that by adjusting the spine, chiropractors can regulate the nerves that travel everywhere else in our body, and thus cure dysfunction. Our theory is that those suggesting this are a bit dysfunctional themselves, and could use a bit of adjustment.

Because of various scope-of-practice issues, as well as the risks of bad chiropractic outcomes being more publicized over the years, more and more states have strict regulations on what chiropractors can do. Ultimately, the chiropractor is still well known for giving your neck and back a good crack. It has been shown that even that sensation can be addictive, so, beware of becoming a crack addict.

60

Dying for Sleep

You might think that sleeping in is good for you, but one study from the medical school of two of the authors—and therefore the study must be great—suggests that sleeping eight hours is associated with a higher death rate than sleeping six to seven hours. This contradicts the widely held belief that humans need eight hours of sleep. Little did we realize when doing our sleep-deprived residencies that our residency directors were actually looking out for our health.

The reason for the increased death rate is unclear, as many other studies show that when individuals do not have the right amount of sleep, their adrenal glands release cortisol, the main stress hormone in the body. Cortisol increases blood sugar, which provides energy; but the hormone also increases abdominal fat, suppresses the immune system, and can increase the risk of developing diabetes and high blood pressure, all of which are associated with a shorter life span. Sleep deprivation while driving or operating heavy machinery is also associated with a severely shortened life span.

So the next time you have a big exam, interview, or presentation in the morning and are debating whether to stay up late the night before, feel free to go ahead and get less sleep. It's clearly good for you in the long run.

Besides, you can sleep when you're dead.

61

Drinking to Improve Thinking

Where do we start?

A majority of students at the University of Southern California might tell you that alcohol is "good" for your health, livens your personality, helps your looks, makes you money, freshens your breath, and improves every aspect of your life. But they probably wouldn't say that it improves brain function, too, would they?

In fact, according to a recent study, the more alcohol the better, up to thirty drinks per week! If there were only a term for people who drank that much. . . .

The theory is that alcohol improves blood flow to the brain, resulting in improved mental functioning. A competing theory is that those who believe this have had a few too many drinks themselves.

As that patient's thinking might suggest, a number of studies have shown a decrease in intelligent thinking from higher alcohol use, and alcohol is known to be toxic to neurons in the brain. The unexpected finding of improved mental functioning with alcohol consumption was found in a population of British civil servants. Perhaps their improved cognitive functioning was due to a decrease in their alcohol use to *only* thirty drinks per week?

Overall, for every study showing health benefits of alcohol, there are many, many more showing harmful effects, including possible liver disease, heart failure, death, and, in the worst-case scenario, man boobs. There may be a temptation to ignore these findings and selectively cite studies that seem to justify excessive drinking. For those who choose this route, take it from the ER doctor who wrote this . . . see you soon!

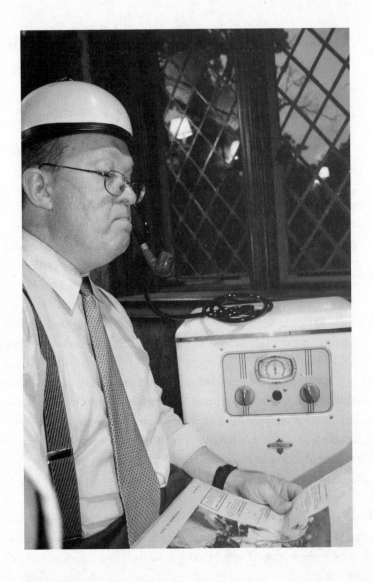

A 1937 Crosley Xervac, hair growth stimulation device.
Credit: Mike Martini, Media Heritage, Inc.

62

Your Mane or
Your Manliness?

For most people, baldness wouldn't make it into the Top Ten Worst Things Ever; that list is more likely to be dominated by Ebola, cancer, dementia, and Kevin Federline's *Playing with Fire* album. Nonetheless, it is a condition that countless men find distressing as they endure taunts like "Mr. Clean," "cue ball," or "chrome dome."

Surprisingly, attempts at curing baldness do not originate in our modern, superficial society. Actually, when it comes to palliating the naturally depilated pate, strange "cures" date back thousands of years. The Ebers Papyrus, which dates to around 1550 BC, includes various treatments for keeping big bad baldness at bay: a concoction of fats from a hippopotamus, a crocodile, a tomcat, a snake, and an ibex; applying porcupine hair boiled in water to the scalp for four days; and consumption of the leg of a female greyhound, sautéed in oil, with a side of donkey hoof. We know what you're thinking: Who has that kind of time?

Options weren't much better a thousand years later when Hippocrates himself, "the father of Western medicine," started having a less hirsute head. His answer: a mixture of opium, horseradish, pigeon droppings, beetroot, and spices applied to the head. We are not sure if that helped with baldness, but wouldn't be surprised if some of his followers tried to smoke each other's heads. Perhaps *that's* where "pothead" originated from?

Fast-forward another thirteen hundred years or so and meet Al-Kindi, a philosopher/doctor from the Baghdad area. He recommended pulverizing a goat's cloven hoofs with vinegar and applying it to the head. Another eleven hundred years or so later, the recommendations in the United States included rubbing kerosene on the head, washing hair with "strong sage tea," applying a mixture of cantharides, capsicum, quinine, and alcohol to the head, and using salt and white oak bark on the head.

And now we must boldly go where many self-respecting balding men dare not, other than Victoria's Secret: the territory of the comb-over and toupee. Reportedly Julius Caesar tried the comb-over, French king Louis XIII popularized the toupee, and George Costanza of *Seinfeld* fame tried both. But those who just can't seem to embrace their inner Michael Jordan or Captain Picard have put far stranger things on their heads. Case in point: the Thermocap, made by the Allied Merke Institute in the 1920s. The idea was to put this helmetlike gadget on your head for fifteen minutes per day and thereby stimulate new hair growth owing to the combination of heat and blue light from the Thermocap. There was also the Xervac, produced in 1936 by the Crosley Corporation, a company that is still around today. This vacuum-like device was supposed to cause hair growth by using suction—just the first of many iterations of the Flowbee.

Some of our follicularly challenged readers may be left wondering if there is any modern, scientific solution for baldness. Well, we imagine not many will choose this option, but, according to a study conducted at Duke University, "eunuchs will not develop baldness if castrated before age 25." So there you have it, dear readers: If you want to have hair, just cut off your junk.

Seriously, don't do that.

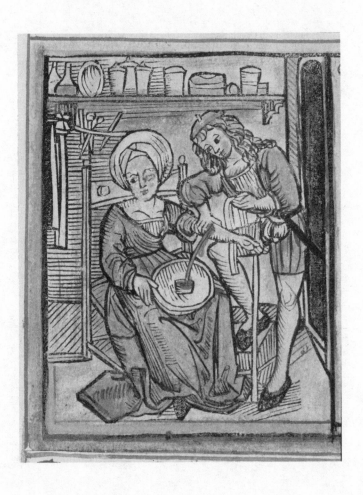

Physician performing bloodletting procedure.
Credit: Private Collection/Archives Charmet/Bridgeman Images.

63

Paging Dr. Dracula

According to Dr. Gilbert R. Seigworth, bloodletting began with ancient Egyptians around 1000 BC and persisted until the end of the nineteenth century. The purpose of bloodletting—deliberately taking blood from the body—was to release the evil spirits from the body and cleanse it—like juice fasting. Dr. Seigworth states: "The early instruments included thorns, pointed sticks and bones, sharp pieces of flint or shell, and even sharply pointed shark's teeth. Miniature bow and arrow devices for bloodletting have been found in South America and New Guinea." One reason bloodletting persisted for so long is that, much like Greek yogurt, kombucha, and chia seeds these days, it was sold as a "cure-all." It was a widely accepted treatment for plague, acne, insanity, herpes, smallpox, pneumonia, epilepsy, gout, leprosy, inflammation, and numerous other conditions.

According to a Canadian medical journal, venesection, or surgical incision of a vein, was the most common method used for bloodletting—other methods included cupping (putting cups on the skin to create suction) and leeching—and it "usually involved the median cubital vein at the elbow, but many different veins could be used. The main instruments for this technique were called lancets and fleams." These instruments were made of ivory, tortoise shells, wood, or various metals.

Some of you might think that nothing like this would happen

today in, as U.S. politicians often like to remind us, "the number one health care system in the world." Right? Actually, the World Health Organization informs us that the U.S. health care system is ranked number thirty-eight, but, thanks to Stephen Colbert, the truthiness of the matter is that we can still believe we're number one! You may be surprised to know that bloodletting—or rather, in its modern form, phlebotomy therapy—is still used at times for a few medical conditions, such as hemochromatosis (too much iron stored in various parts of the body), polycythemia vera (excessive blood cells), and porphyria cutanea tarda (abnormal iron metabolism).

However, there may be more indications on the horizon. A recent medical article mentions that "Two sessions of bloodletting were enough to improve blood pressure and markers of cardiovascular disease" in obese people with metabolic syndrome. Take-home point: Screw diet and exercise—bring on the sharks' teeth and mini bows and arrows!

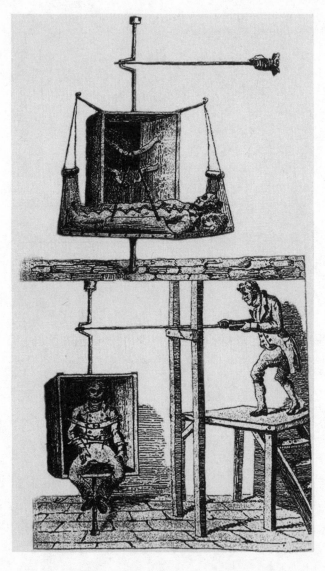

A bed and chair designed specifically to provide "spinning therapy." Obtained from: oewf.org/en/2012/11/space-medicine-inhale-rusty/coxs-chair-kopie_small-2/. Public Domain.

64

Hurling at High Speed

The British band Dead or Alive had a hit with their 1985 song "You Spin Me Round (Like a Record)." Roller skaters of the 1980s quickly adopted the song as their anthem and literally spun around in circles to the blasting tune. The history of medicine also has a chapter that involved patients being spun right round—often involuntarily and at high speeds—leaving them not dead, per se, but likely not very glad to be alive.

One of the original proponents of the idea behind "spinning therapy," aka "centrifuge therapy" and "spinning chair therapy," was Erasmus Darwin, a physician and the grandfather of Charles Darwin. Erasmus thought that a "rotative couch" could induce sleep in those with mental illness, thereby improving their mental condition. Others proposed that spinning would help to reduce congestion in the brain, which was thought to produce many psychiatric symptoms. However, physician Joseph Mason Cox took the idea to the next level.

In the late 1700s, he designed a special chair—which he humbly (and probably without much foresight) called Cox's chair. The Cox chair enabled him to spin patients more easily on a vertical axis than a regular chair allowed. The chair, which paved the way for spinning beds, also included leather straps and straitjackets to secure patients and keep them from falling out or maintaining dignity.

Now, anyone who has ever been on the spinning-teacup ride at

Disneyland, or anyone who has reached the age of five, knows that spinning fast is more likely to result in nausea than a nap or time travel. Even the astute Dr. Cox noted this: "One of the most constant effects of swinging is a greater or less degree of vertigo, attended by pallor, nausea, and vomiting; and frequently by the evacuation of the contents of the bladder."

Nonetheless, he advocated for the chair: "After a few circumvolutions, I have witnessed the soothing lulling effects, when the mind has become tranquilized, and the body quiescent; a degree of vertigo has often followed, and this been succeeded by the most refreshing slumbers."

But wait! There's more!

Undoubtedly, the staff who had to clean up the vomitus and "contents of the bladder" probably did not appreciate the Cox chair, which fell out of favor as a psychiatric treatment in the early nineteenth century. Still, Cox's invention and other versions based on it were later used in studies of motion, vertigo, and vestibular function. Some time later, everyone completely forgot everything they had learned and made this a ride at the county fair.

"Spinning therapy" is no longer used today, and a Cox chair has an entirely different meaning. But if you still want to experience vertigo, pallor, nausea, and vomiting, you can either fork over $100 for a Disneyland ticket . . . or $2.48 for a can of Spam.

65

Possibly a Posset for Parity?

Ask any woman who has ever been pregnant and she will likely confirm that receiving unsolicited and contradictory advice regarding the pregnancy/labor/baby is the norm and often annoying as hell, especially when the advice comes from men. One of the most controversial topics is use of alcohol during pregnancy. Some people argue that a small amount of alcohol is just fine, whereas others like the idea about as much as Kanye West likes sharing . . . anything. Regardless of how one feels about it, one question that also comes up frequently is the effect of alcohol on the induction of labor. (Which is a fair enough question, seeing as how alcohol seems to induce many other things, like drunk texts and the sex that likely led to the pregnancy in the first place.)

The prevalent "common sense" belief is that a glass of wine can help to induce labor by making the pregnant woman feel more relaxed. However, as reported on a parenting website, alcohol can actually have just the opposite effect. Two physicians, who specialize in obstetrics and gynecology, point out that alcohol can limit or stop contractions by relaxing the uterus. In fact, there was a time (1970s or so) when it was used to stop preterm labor.

As much as we wish this would settle the matter once and for all, alas, science, like childbirth, is a messy process, and scientific consensus on this issue is far from clear. For instance, a Danish study looked at the risk of preterm delivery for women consuming alcohol during their pregnancies. According to the authors, their study found an increased risk of preterm deliveries associated with the consumption of seven or more drinks per week. The authors also acknowledge the use of alcohol to avoid premature labor in the past, but its use has not been supported by clinical trials. (Although, if the couple had avoided alcohol nine months prior, that probably could've been the ultimate avoidance of premature labor.) They argue that alcohol can induce preterm delivery via increasing the production of prostaglandins. This last assertion is supported by another study, conducted in pregnant mice, which were given alcohol and found to have an increased level of a prostaglandin.

Given that the controversy over this issue still remains, the value of this study remains somewhat dubious in our eyes. But the visual of cute little secondhand drunk baby mice getting into bar fights is pretty priceless!

Sidebar: Something not so cute to imagine: baby mice wine. Apparently some people in China and Korea drink a "health tonic" made by dropping newly born baby mice into a vat of rice wine and letting the whole thing ferment. At some later time, the imbibers drink the "tonic" and eat the baby mice.

We'll take that tequila worm any day.

66

Parsley, Sage, Rosemary, and Thyme

This is the part of the book where we sound like we're about to make light of a very serious and difficult topic—termination of pregnancy—but we are actually going to highlight a rather unusual abortifacient.

The substance we are referring to is apiol, which is found in parsley (as well as celery leaf) and is also called parsley camphor. A scientist, Heinrich Christoph Link, reportedly discovered it in 1715. It took more than a hundred years before it was found—by accident—that it could induce menstruation in many women having irregular menstrual cycles. Reportedly, apiol was initially used to treat some people sick with malaria. Although it didn't work for malaria, some of these patients, who also had amenorrhea (absence of menstruation), began having regular menstrual cycles as a side effect of the apiol. And the men they lived with rejoiced, and God saw that it was good.

Apiol quickly became popular for menstrual irregularity, and later also as an abortifacient. Per a recent report, it "increases the tone and strength of miometral [uterine muscle] contraction, reduces the tone of vessels and causes necrosis [death] of placental tissue." Apiol, in many forms, was used widely in the United States before the era of safer, medical abortions, especially because it did not require a prescription. By one estimate, at one time about half of all voluntary abortions were carried out through the use of apiol.

According to the same source, "The lowest dose of apiol that seems to be necessary to induce abortion is 0.9g taken for eight consecutive days." However, it is not benign and can cause serious side effects, including liver and kidney damage, severe blood loss, abdominal pain, vomiting, coma, and brain damage. The medical journal *Lancet* has even reported death resulting from an attempt to use apiol to induce abortion.

Although discovery of apiol is relatively new, parsley itself has been purported to cause abortion for centuries, going back to the era of Hippocrates (about 400 BC) and buffet tables everywhere. Parsley, celery leaf, and many other plants have been used by women for millennia to terminate pregnancies. As if America needed another excuse to pick pizza over salad. But seriously, eating a small amount of parsley or celery leaf does not pose any risk, so please don't tell your significant other that you are avoiding your veggies on doctors' orders.

As for the rather controversial topic of unintended pregnancy and abortion, no matter where you fall on that spectrum, we think you will agree with Dorothy Parker's sentiment: "It serves me right for putting all my eggs in one bastard."

67

Finally, a Medical Reason to *Not* Exercise

Ben-Gay, the sports cream used to treat muscle and joint pains, gets about as much respect as Tom Cruise in any movie after *Jerry Maguire*. Jokes about "old people having a Ben-Gay smell," although unfortunate and ageist, have been around for decades. Even the indie band Magnapop, who reportedly named their album *Rubbing Doesn't Help* for a Ben-Gay slogan, did not manage to make Ben-Gay sound hip and cool. Nonetheless, given that it's been around for more than a hundred years, our guess is that it must work for a lot of people. However, this does not mean that excessive Ben-Gay use goes without side effects.

In fact, in June 2007 Fox News reported an unusual and rare case of a death attributed (at least partly) to the overuse of Ben-Gay. Unlike most Fox News stories, this story is unfortunately true. A seventeen-year-old track star was found dead, and an autopsy revealed that her blood contained lethal amounts of methyl salicylate, one of the active ingredients of Ben-Gay (and other sports creams). Per report, she was using Ben-Gay, among other products. Per NBC News, Dr. Thomas Kearney, a professor of clinical pharmacology at the University of California at San Francisco, added, "Topical application of methyl salicylate can be hazardous if it is smeared over 40 percent of the body, if someone has a skin condition or if another medication interacts negatively with the products."

Though direct methyl salicylate toxicity from topical creams is unlikely, it is important to keep in mind that the risk of toxicity is increased under certain conditions. For instance, using a heating pad (which melts the cream and also opens up the pores on the body) and taking oral salicylate products, like aspirin or Pepto-Bismol, while at the same time using Bengay can Far and Away (get it!?) increase the risk of overdosing on salicylate.

Even rigorous exercising can increase the Risky Business (we're almost done), as it reportedly can act like a heating pad; in fact, this is thought to have happened in the case above. So whatever you do, please do not engage in heavy-duty Tom Cruise couch jumping while using any sports cream with methyl salicylate. Even if it doesn't lead to any toxicity, it'll be Mission Impossible to be taken seriously by anyone after that!

Also, Cocktail.

68

Poor Pooh Bear

Warning: Lovers of Winnie-the-Pooh, Baloo, and Fozzie might want to grab a tissue box and take a Xanax before reading further, because the following is quite upsetting.

In traditional Chinese medicine, bear bile plays a big role. This gastrointestinal goop is thought to treat numerous conditions. According to Ben Kavoussi, the book *Chinese Herbal Medicine: Materia Medica* includes "trauma, sprains, fractures, hemorrhoids, conjunctivitis, severe hepatitis, high fever, convulsions, and delirium" as conditions purportedly treated by bear bile. In addition, it is claimed that bear bile can reduce gallstones, improve eyesight, and help fight off the flu, and is helpful for hangovers due to excessive alcohol consumption. Although there is little evidence that it actually works, it has become more popular recently, especially as more people now have insurance coverage for medicines made from bear bile. Thank you, Obamacare.

Unfortunately, the process of obtaining the bile from bears—usually Asiatic black bears, a threatened species—is extremely cruel and painful. Bears are often captured as cubs in the wild, or, less frequently, raised in captivity. Bile is usually extracted two to three times a day by inserting a large needle into the animal, or surgically implanting a tube in the bear so it can be "milked." According to the Humane Society, the process is very painful for the bears and they often chew their paws because of the trauma and anxiety induced by the procedure. Bears are kept in small cages, typically so small that they are not able to turn around. As some bears can live for twenty years or so, they are subjected to this horrible procedure for a long time (although many succumb to infections and tumors/cancers brought on by repeated "milkings"). We told you to get tissues.

The active ingredient in bear bile is thought to be ursodeoxycholic acid (UA). According to Dr. David Garshelis of the United Nations International Union for Conservation of Nature, some studies do show that UA can help treat specific types of liver disorders, such as primary biliary cirrhosis; however, no scientific consensus exists. Fortunately, UA is readily available in synthetic, cruelty-free form. Nevertheless, traditionalists eschew the synthetic version and argue that the "natural" bile is more potent. *The New York Times* reported that Fang Shuting, chairman of the China Association of Traditional Chinese Medicine, went as far as to suggest that "bears enjoy the process, which he likened to turning on a tap. 'Natural, easy and without pain,' he said. 'After they're done, the bears can even play happily outside.'"

We think if Baloo heard that, he'd surely like to stick a prickly pear up someone's gall bladder and ask him if he enjoyed the process!

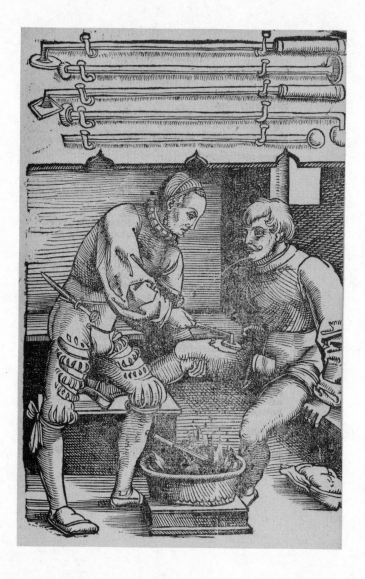

A heated piece of metal being applied to the wound, likely to stop heavy bleeding.
Credit: Wellcome Library, London. Obtained from: Creative Commons by 4.0.

69

And It Burns, Burns, Burns, the Ring of Fire . . .

Stedman's Medical Dictionary defines "cauterization" as "cutting the skin or other tissues by means of heat, cold, electric current, ultrasound, or caustic chemicals." The process of cautery has been used historically to stop bleeding, remove abnormal growth, and prevent infections. However, early forms of cautery were quite different from their modern equivalents.

Probably the first form of cautery consisted of heating stones and applying them to the bleeding sites to stop the bleeding (the high temperature would cause the blood to coagulate). We're guessing that this was as painful as it sounds, so it's not surprising that stones were replaced by heated metal. Andreas Vesalius, considered by many to be the father of modern human anatomy, was a big proponent of cautery. He proposed two methods: "One is performed by fire, whether by charcoal or by a hot iron. . . . The other method is the use of medicaments which possess the strength of burning." Of course, if the patient refused these options, there was always the backup plan: applying hot oil—and not in a fun, flirtatious, "Hey, can you put some oil on my back" kind of way. Maybe we are just glass-half-empty types, but this hot-oil method does not sound like a big improvement.

On the other hand, it could be worse . . . much worse. According to the French physician Ambroise Paré (1510–1590), another royal surgeon shared with Paré his recipe for healing gunshot wounds. The recipe called for boiling two puppies in the oil of lilies, adding one pound of earthworms, straining the mixture through a napkin, and adding some herbs to make a balm.

Fortunately for pup and canine lovers everywhere, the development of electrocautery appears to have been a major step forward. As reported by Dr. Nader M. Massarweh and others in the *Journal of American College of Surgeons*, the first use of electricity in surgery was in 1900 by a French physician, Joseph Rivere. The modern electrocautery instruments used today are based on an earlier version developed by an American scientist, William Bovie. Nevertheless, a body of studies suggests that some electric cautery may actually increase the risk of infection by causing tissue damage and making it easier for bacteria to grow.

We're still thinking about the poor puppies, so we're just going to stop here, go make a donation to the ASPCA, and call it a night.

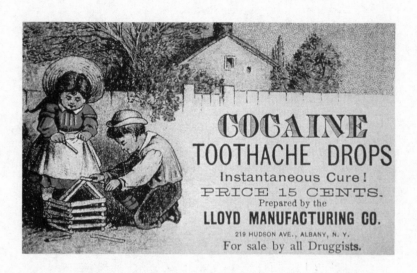

An advertisement for cocaine toothache drops from the late 1800s.
Credit: Science Source.

70

Snow in Your Nose

The Beat poet Allen Ginsberg reportedly wrote, "Nobody saves America by sniffing cocaine / Jiggling yr knees blankeyed in the rain / When it snows in yr nose you catch cold in yr brain." Though the Beats certainly had a reputation for heavy drug use, many readers might be surprised to learn how many respected figures in the past not only used cocaine but recommended its use to others.

One of the most famous proponents of cocaine was Dr. Sigmund Freud, one of the founders of psychoanalysis and the unlikely originator of "your mom" jokes. Not only did he use cocaine for years, he also recommended it to colleagues and patients as a treatment for depression, sexual impotence, and (ironically) addiction. In fact, one of his first medical publications was a tract about cocaine called *Über Coca*, published in 1884. In it Freud argued that "cocaine was so effective at treating morphine and alcohol abuse that 'inebriate asylums can be entirely dispensed with.'"

Although Freud may have been overly optimistic in his assessment of the health benefits of cocaine, it is true that the source of cocaine, the coca leaf (*Erythroxylum coca*), has been chewed by many Peruvians (as it is native to Peru) to ward off fatigue and hunger. Cocaine was isolated from the coca leaf in 1859 by Albert Niemann in Germany. The original Coca-Cola, concocted in 1886, contained a small amount of cocaine, which is thought to have boosted its popularity. Though Freud may not have been a household name in the United States back then, certainly the high profile of cocaine's other admirers helped to popularize it.

For example, William S. Halsted, the famous surgeon who devised the radical mastectomy for breast cancer and was one of the founders of the Johns Hopkins Hospital, also experimented with cocaine to study its topical anesthetic properties. He injected cocaine into the nerves of many colleagues, medical students, and patients to show that it could block pain. His general idea was correct, but, much like a comic-book character in the 1960s, he also received such injections as part of these experiments—and eventually he became addicted to cocaine. And just so you don't think doctors were the only ones excited by what would eventually become the nose candy of choice in 1980s America, famous people outside the medical field also reportedly touted the benefits of cocaine, including Thomas Edison and Sarah Bernhardt.

If all this seems a quaint, distant past, think again. As of this writing (2015), "The American Academy of Otolaryngology-Head and Neck Surgery, Inc., considers cocaine to be a valuable anesthetic and vasoconstricting agent when used as part of the treatment of a patient by a physician. No other single drug combines the anesthetic and vasoconstricting properties of cocaine." By causing vasoconstriction (narrowing blood vessels), cocaine can decrease swelling and blood loss. And due to its fast-onset action as an anesthetic (causing numbness), it can decrease pain.

So some might argue that, in light of all the problems now being associated with soda, cocaine just may have been the healthiest—or at least the most useful—ingredient in it. We can almost see the newly minted Facebook petition to bring it back.

71

Aspire to Respire, but Avoid to Not Expire

You would think that a plant known by names such as "devil's weed," "hell's bells," "stinkweed," "pricklyburr," "devil's snare," "devil's trumpet," and so on, would be clearly avoided by most, especially the medical establishment. But when it comes to *Datura stramonium*, more commonly known as Jimson weed in the United States, it's not that simple.

To be sure, Jimson weed is associated with serious side effects when used. (Parts of the plant are usually ingested or smoked by those looking to get "high" from it.) A recent search of medical databases revealed more than one hundred published articles referencing reports of Jimson weed toxicity. The Centers for Disease Control and Prevention (CDC) clearly warns on its website, "All parts of the Jimson weed plant are poisonous, containing the alkaloids atropine, hyoscyamine, and scopolamine." These alkaloids are classified as anticholinergics and do have genuine medicinal applications when used appropriately. For example, these alkaloids have been used to control nausea/vomiting and stabilize the heart rate. However, toxicity from these substances results in symptoms like dry mucous membranes, difficulty swallowing and speaking, blurred vision, hyperthermia, confusion, agitation, hallucinations, urinary retention, seizures, coma, and, rarely, death. (Same symptoms you'd get if you watched *The Bachelor* or *The Bachelorette* for a while.)

However, atropine has also been used to treat asthma for a long time. Although it's no longer the first treatment of choice for most people in the United States, many patients still take it. So it's not surprising that in India, in the traditional Ayurvedic medicine, Jimson weed has been used for centuries to help with asthma. Likewise, in Africa, Jimson weed has a long history of use as a treatment for asthma.

This practice eventually also spread to Europe and the United States. And in one of medicine's you-just-can't-make-this-up ironies, Jimson weed was actually smoked—initially in pipes, later as cigarettes—to help asthmatics both obtain quick relief and look cooler in the halls at school. In fact, according to the *Medical Times and Gazette*, in 1875 a Jimson weed-containing product called the Cigares de Joy was recommended to "cure asthma, wheezing, and winter cough" and advertised as being so "harmless in its action, [that] it may be safely smoked by ladies and children." We know now, of course, that smoking can trigger asthma. But given the presence and action of atropine, it is quite likely that some people with asthma did notice an improvement in their breathing.

So in summary, a little bit and you might no longer wheeze; but overdo it, and you might no longer breathe.

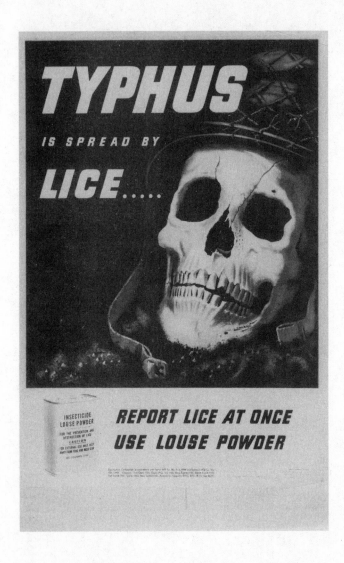

A historical poster warning about the dangers of lice.
Credit: Otis Historical Archives. Obtained from: Creative Commons by 2.0.

72

Liquidating Lousy Lice

DDT, less easily called dichlorodiphenyltrichloroethane, is infamous as the insecticide that American biologist Rachel Carson discussed in her book *Silent Spring* and linked to various negative effects on human and animal health. More specifically, she argued that DDT and other pesticides were linked to cancer and threatened fish and birds. Many historians give much credit to her book for inspiring the environmental movement and eventually leading to a wide ban on DDT and the chemical's inclusion in a Joni Mitchell song.

However, the history and usefulness of DDT is more complex than the series finale of *Lost*. Reportedly, DDT was first synthesized in 1874 by German chemist Othmar Zeidler, but not used until 1939, when the Swiss scientist Paul Hermann Müller synthesized it again. He also discovered its insect-killing properties, which eventually led to its use in killing typhus-carrying lice. (He was later given a Nobel Prize for his discovery.) With louse infestation a major concern at the onset of World War II, a team of American entomologists discovered that DDT was quite effective against the louse and other pests.

As documented by Naomi Baumslag in the book *Murderous Medicine: Nazi Doctors, Human Experimentation, and Typhus*, DDT "was first used on a large scale to control a typhus epidemic in Naples, Italy, in 1943, where the U.S. military made history by bringing the epidemic quickly under control." Unfortunately, even though it was initially recommended solely for delousing and malaria control, gradually DDT was used very widely and entered the food chain of various animals and fish, as documented in *Silent Spring*. On a good note, the subsequent DDT ban is thought to have significantly helped in the recovery of the bald eagle and peregrine falcon populations.

We would happily take that eagle—bald or not—any day over a louse with a full head of hair.

73

A Cup Should Not Go Up

Howard Schultz, the CEO of Starbucks, once quipped, "Starbucks represents something beyond a cup of coffee." If only he knew that for some people, the "beyond" in this case is the behind.

A lot of us drink coffee. Starbucks is a household name, and even more "hipster" coffees like Stumptown and Blue Bottle are celebrated in major newspapers like the *The New York Times*. But in certain "alternative medicine" circles the coffee enema is quite popular as well.

The concept of the coffee enema appears to be about a hundred years old. *The Merck Manual of Diagnosis and Therapy*, one of the most widely sold medical texts, mentioned coffee enemas until its 1972 edition. In the 1920s, Max Gerson, a German American physician, recommended coffee enemas as a potential cure for cancer. More recently, Suzy Cohen, who calls herself "America's Most Trusted Pharmacist," claimed that "coffee enemas may help relieve constipation, insomnia and cognitive problems; they may eliminate (or control) parasites, candida and other pathogens (without disrupting intestinal flora). . . . These enemas may allow for relaxation, a better mood, more energy, refreshing sleep and greater mental clarity."

Many proponents of coffee enemas believe in the theory of autointoxication. Based on medical concepts derived in ancient Egypt and Greece—and largely disproven by modern medicine—adherents of autointoxication believe that over time, fecal matter in the colon can harbor harmful toxins, bacteria, and/or parasites, which can cause poor health, including symptoms like fatigue, chronic pain, headaches, irritability, anxiety, depression, and loss of appetite. However, as pointed out by Scott Gavura on his *Science-Based Medicine* blog, there are numerous, potentially serious side effects of coffee enemas. Various medical papers have documented issues, including the introduction of bacteria into the bloodstream (which can be deadly if not treated quickly), rectal perforation, and electrolyte abnormalities. In fact, the *Journal of the American Medical Association* published an article in October 1980 with the title "Deaths Related to Coffee Enemas," which was—unsurprisingly— about the deaths of two patients related to coffee enemas.

Our bottom-line recommendation? Keep coffee away from your bottom—it's Stumptown and Blue Bottle, not Rumptown and Brown Bottle.

74

Lettin' Go Lentigo

Doctors generally ignore freckles, as they tend to be benign with no medical consequences (but those same doctors, especially dermatologists, will call them "lentigos" to impress their patients). Likewise, most people with freckles probably don't think much about them on a daily basis. Others may even find them cute or sexy, especially if the freckles happen to be attached to a famous model or celebrity (e.g., Emma Stone). On the other hand, the desire to remove freckles is also ancient, as are the slew of "recommended" treatments and cures to do so.

According to the ancient Indian system of Ayurvedic medicine, freckles could be removed by using pastes consisting of ingredients like banana, mint, lemon, salt, honey, turmeric, buttermilk, uva ursi—a type of berry—and other herbs and spices. These pastes probably also made a good smoothie. To this day, modern Ayurvedic practitioners recommend these treatments. Traditional Chinese medicine has its own theories regarding what causes freckles and how to remove them. Dr. Yim Yiu-kin, a registered Chinese medicine practitioner, notes, "According to theories in Chinese Medicine, liver has a close reciprocal relationship with one's emotions. If one's emotion is unstable, it will affect normal functioning of liver, leading to an increased chance of developing freckles on the face." Treatments recommended by Dr. Yiu-kin include: black fungus and red date soup; a mixture of mung beans, adzuki beans, and lily buds; and a drink made up of milk, soy milk, and ground walnuts and sesame seeds.

The tradition of such remedies in the United States is not nearly as old, of course, given the relatively young age of the country. Nevertheless, as freckled individuals make up a significant portion of the population, many remedies have been historically suggested. The instructions for one of these say to "take one half teacupful of rain water and two teaspoonfuls of powdered borax, and with this wash the parts twice a day. This is a never-failing remedy for removing freckles of people possessing certain textures of skin." Other remedies in the same list were made up of English mustard, lemon juice, sour milk, sugar, glycerine, and "the milky juice of the stem of the dandelion."

Just in case any of our readers are inclined to mock these old "medical treatments" as being obviously outdated and implausible, we just want to point out that even now such remedies are easily and commonly found on the modern Oracle of Medical Wisdom, the Internet. For instance, a quick search turns up these items being recommended to remove freckles: lemon juice, sour cream, honey, papaya, onion, buttermilk, castor oil, horseradish, eggplant, sesame seeds, cucumber, almond oil, tomato juice, olive oil, strawberries, jojoba oil, orange peel, vitamin E oil.

We would love to discuss this topic further, but for some reason we have an overwhelming desire to fix a snack.

75

Hashing Out
Headbanging Hazards

Readers of a certain age might remember a show on MTV called *Headbangers Ball*. (Readers of a different—i.e., younger—age may be surprised to learn that MTV ever played music. They may be even more surprised to learn that the "M" in MTV actually stood for Music, not Monotonous.) Anyway, although the popularity of the show has fluctuated throughout the years, headbanging to metal, hard rock, and other genres of music has always had its share of fans. And, no doubt, many of our readers fall into this category. So, uncool as it may be, for the sake of our readers' health, we feel it necessary to point out some of the potential downsides of headbanging.

Cue the ceremonious record scratch.

A quick definition for our readers who are more into John Denver than Judas Priest. The *Oxford English Dictionary* defines head-banging as "a style of dancing, typically to heavy metal or hard rock music, involving vigorous and rhythmic nodding or shaking of the head." It certainly sounds harmless, especially when compared with actually banging one's head into a stuccoed surface. However, according to a study published in the *BMJ*, two researchers from Australia found that "an average head banging song has a tempo of about 146 beats per minute, which is predicted to cause mild head injury when the range of motion is greater than 75°. At higher tempos and greater ranges of motion there is a risk of neck injury."

Granted, this was published in the yearly "joke" issue of *BMJ*, but there is other anecdotal evidence. For instance, as accurately reported by the *Scientific American* joke blog, "a 15-year-old drummer in his neighborhood band suffered an aneurysm in his cervical vertebral artery, according to a 1991 case report in the journal *Pediatric Neurosurgery*, and Evanescence guitarist Terry Balsamo had a stroke three years ago that his docs blamed on his head-banging tendencies." A more recent case, published in the medical journal *Lancet* (not in a "joke" issue), involved a man who developed a head bleed after attending a concert and headbanging to the music. The authors, all German doctors, concluded, "We assume that headbanging, with its brisk forward and back acceleration and deceleration forces, led to rupturing of bridging veins causing haemorrhage into the subdural space."

So if you are a headbanging fan, what should you do? Well, you can switch to Celine Dion, but frankly we'd rather have a subdural hematoma than subject our brain to how passionate she is about her heart going on. Fortunately, the authors of the *BMJ* study recommend another option: "To minimise the risk of head and neck injury, head bangers should decrease their range of head and neck motion, head bang to slower tempo songs by replacing heavy metal with adult oriented rock, only head bang to every second beat, or use personal protective equipment."

Take-home point, as the authors also point out: Headbanging like Beavis is safer than headbanging like Butthead (which should resolve, once and for all, the great debate as to which one of them is cooler).

An old advertisement recommending heroin as a cure for various maladies.
Credit: Wellcome Library, London. Obtained from: Creative Commons by 4.0.

76

Heroin: The All-Time Addictive, Snorting, Injecting, Smoking, Disorienting, Constipating, So-You-Can-Throw-It-All-Away Medicine

We doubt there are many readers who have not heard about the terrible dangers of heroin, thanks to HBO and various installments of *CSI*. According to the National Institute of Drug Abuse, "in 2011, 4.2 million Americans aged 12 or older (or 1.6 percent) had used heroin at least once in their lives. It is estimated that about 23 percent of individuals who use heroin become dependent on it." Even on a more pop-culture level, the highly acclaimed TV show *The Wire* and the ever-cool Velvet Underground song "Heroin" highlight the consequences of using heroin. However, there was a time when heroin was actively promoted as a nonaddictive treatment for—of all things!—cough.

Heroin, also known as diacetylmorphine, was first reportedly synthesized in England by a chemist named Charles Romley Alder Wright. However, he did not do much with it. About twenty years later, Felix Hoffman, working at the pharmaceutical company Bayer, independently synthesized heroin while trying to make codeine. (Hate when that happens.)

Bayer claimed that heroin was nonaddictive and started selling it in 1898, encouraging its use for treating asthma, bronchitis, and tuberculosis. It was also used to treat morphine addiction initially (even though heroin is converted to morphine in the body when ingested). However, among heroin addicts, ingestion is not the preferred route because when heroin is used intravenously it is multiple times more potent than morphine and produces a greater "high."

Of course, within months after Bayer started selling heroin, it became obvious that although heroin did indeed help with cough, it was highly addictive. (Whooooops.) However, it wasn't until 1913 that Bayer stopped selling it, and as late as 1912 Bayer was promoting it in Europe as a cough medicine for children. In the United States, the FDA required a prescription for heroin starting in 1914, and eventually banned it, in 1924. It resurfaced in the 1980s in breakfast-cereal form, under the title of Cap'n Crunch. (Just kidding.)

Fortunately, we know better now, so no more heroin cough syrup. Unfortunately, we are stuck with cough syrups that, although not addictive, also don't seem to do anything except leave us feeling groggy and heavy-headed the next day.

77

Halting Harassing Hiccups

Hiccups, which are involuntary contractions of the diaphragm (the muscle between your chest area and abdomen) followed by vocal-cord closure, are one of the mild annoyances of life that all of us put up with—usually for a few minutes every few months or so—and then forget all about. Thankfully, most of us are not like Charles Osborne, who started hiccupping in 1922, while attempting to weigh a hog before slaughtering it, and continued to hiccup for the next . . . sixty-eight years (for a total of 430 million hiccups!).

Nonetheless, even a brief duration of hiccups can be annoying, and occasionally, somewhat painful. So there is certainly an interest in treating them, although there does not appear to be a perfect treatment that works in all cases. On the plus side, some of the purported treatments are highly amusing. In fact, there is an old *Calvin and Hobbes* cartoon in which Hobbes quips, "I think most hiccup cures were really invented for the amusement of the patient's friends."

So true when we consider the following list.

Of course, all of us have heard of folk remedies like standing on one's head, drinking a glass of water upside down, being frightened by someone, holding one's breath, and breathing into a bag. Other American traditional remedies: placing cassia oil on the tongue, or trying camphor, limewater, soda, cold water, ice, snuff, or ice cream. In England, spitting on the forefinger of the right hand and making a cross on the front of the left shoe while saying the Lord's Prayer backward was thought to be effective. The Romans made it much easier: Hold the left thumb in the right hand. Norwegians recommended swallowing a spoonful of white sugar and letting the granules trickle down the back of the throat, whereas the Greeks advised applying a mixture of honey, coriander, and pepper to the tongue for a minute. The Vikings, of course, had to go with something a bit more painful: pulling the tongue forward while slowly counting to one hundred. The Chinese recommended rubbing the roof of the mouth with a cotton swab, as well as acupuncture. The Spanish believed in sprinkling cayenne pepper into vinegar, adding flour, and applying the paste to the diaphragm (sounds like the beginning of a tapas recipe to us). The Swedes, never afraid to look silly, recommended holding one's breath, pinching the thumbs and pinky fingers together, and moving one's arms around in circles.

Some of these interesting remedies have lived into the modern era. But we also have more mundane, yet more effective, treatments, such as the medications chlorpromazine (approved by the FDA for hiccups), gabapentin, baclofen, carvedilol, metoclopramide, and various others. Nerve blockades and nerve ablations are also valid options for some patients.

Hopefully, you will never need to consider any real treatment for hiccups. But please do keep in mind that hiccups that go on for days to months can be due to serious medical issues like strokes, tumors, inflammation, kidney problems, brain injury, etc.

We almost forgot to mention one of the more common causes of hiccups: alcohol. So you may be wondering if drinking alcohol from the wrong side of the glass can prevent/treat hiccups. We are actually actively researching this question by consuming appropriately large quantities of good microbrews. If you would like to contribute to this worthy scientific investigation, please feel free to make a donation via our publisher! Just kidding.

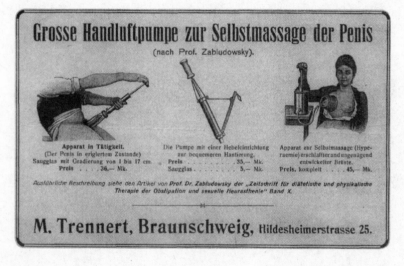

78

The Importance of Impotence

The topic of impotence and its purported treatments is so huge that we doubt anybody could rise to the challenge (get it?) of covering it adequately to satisfy everyone (zing!). But we do want to highlight some rather bizarre and fascinating practices from the past. An excellent source is the book *Impotence: A Cultural History* by Angus McLaren. The author reports that numerous plants have been thought to have aphrodisiac properties, including the leek, garlic, turpentine tree, asparagus, Cyprian reed, clematis, xiphium root, etc. Of course, some followers of the Atkins diet had their own list: snakes, wolves, goats, lizards, sparrows, starfish, genitalia of roosters, and even the ever-popular Spanish fly (which is actually a beetle, and rather toxic). Herbs have been used for centuries to "cure" impotence. In China, ginseng was/is explicitly recommended for this purpose. Other herbs used for this purpose include strychnine, yohimbe, damiana, and cannabis.

Eventually, surgeons also started offering their services to cure impotence. As reported by Dr. Chris Iliades, the first surgical treatment for erectile dysfunction was in 1873 in Italy when a surgeon "successfully treated ED by blocking veins that drained blood away from a penile erection." This success appears to have inspired a bit of overconfidence, as in the early 1900s testicles taken from various sources, like monkeys, human cadavers, goats, boars, and deer, were implanted into impotent men with the idea of curing them. This didn't do much to cure the impotence, but probably did lead to some awkward moments when the recipient of such a transplant took off his clothes for the first time with a new potential partner. Usually, you ask the other party before introducing toys. At any rate, other treatment options included applying electricity to the penis, implants of small metal rods, and using splints to stiffen the penis. Not surprisingly, none of them worked very well.

In 1998, Viagra became the first oral medication to be approved by the U.S. Food and Drug Administration to treat erectile dysfunction. Despite having Bob Dole as its spokesperson, Viagra became the fastest-selling pharmaceutical in history. For the simple reason that it actually works much better than gobbling up goat genitalia . . . and is less awkward than using a penile pump or penile injection, which had been the most often used options prior to Viagra but are just so bulky to travel with. . . .

We hope all those still engaging in eating rhino horns and tiger penises (driving both species to the verge of extinction) start thinking with their right head and reach for the blue pill. If it can get Bob Dole some action, it must be potent!

79

When the Treatment Is
Worse Than the Disease

Usually if a medical procedure has more than one name, one is generally better than the others. However, here is a case in which we can't decide which of two names is worse: insulin coma therapy (ICT) or insulin shock therapy. Regardless, both names describe a terrible and dangerous procedure used by many psychiatrists, especially in the 1940s and 1950s. Reports suggest that Dr. Manfred Sakel, a European psychiatrist, first used it in Vienna and Berlin. An American psychiatrist, Dr. Joseph Wortis, observed Dr. Sakel practice it and introduced it to the United States.

The idea behind insulin coma therapy was to inject insulin in patients with schizophrenia to initially induce hypoglycemia (low blood sugar), and to eventually induce coma. (Because it's not a party unless everyone is miserable?) Giving patients intravenous glucose would terminate the coma. At times, although not always, hypoglycemia would result in seizures. While there were many reports of psychotic patients being helped, how this procedure resulted in improvement in psychosis was never fully explained. Dr. Max Fink, the head of the insulin coma unit at the Hillside Hospital in Glen Oaks, Queens, New York, from 1952 to 1958, described the treatments as "unpleasant and dangerous. They were given without anesthesia. The ICT mortality rate varied from 1% to 10% of patients treated. Prolonged coma, in which the patient did not respond to the administration of glucose, was a constant threat." In the 1950s, Dr. Harold Bourne and others published multiple papers, in the British journal *Lancet*, arguing against ICT as a valid and helpful treatment for schizophrenia.

However, it appears that at least in some patients there was an improvement with ICT. The most famous example is probably John Nash, the American mathematician and Nobel laureate, who was diagnosed with schizophrenia and portrayed in the movie *A Beautiful Mind*. In 1961, he was treated with ICT for six weeks and reportedly improved enough that he was able to work for about a year. Nonetheless, by the 1970s ICT was no longer being used in the United States and most other countries—a fate we wish had also befallen ABBA.

80

I'd Rather Have a Bottle in Front of Me Than a Frontal Lobotomy

Regardless of the debate over who originally said the above, for the record, we agree wholeheartedly. Which is not to discount the interesting history of lobotomy, or leukotomy, as it is also known. But let's start at the beginning.

Evidence suggests that some sort of cranial or psychosurgery has been practiced for centuries, but the "modern" lobotomy was popularized by Egas Moniz, a Portuguese neurologist. As reported by PBS, Moniz thought that some mental illnesses were the result of "an abnormal sort of stickiness in nerve cells, causing neural impulses to get stuck." In 1935, Moniz drilled holes in the skulls of some of his patients suffering from illnesses like schizophrenia, mania, depression, and anxiety, and Moniz injected alcohol into their frontal lobes. And you thought a keg stand was hardcore. Later, instead of injecting alcohol, he began cutting parts of the frontal lobes with an instrument he designed, the leukotome (basically, a loop of wire that could be rotated to create a circular lesion). In 1936 he published the results, claiming that his subjects had improved dramatically. Self-reporting for the win! His article was well received, and soon the practice spread to other countries, despite some serious side effects from the procedure (e.g., apathy, dullness, incontinence, and personality changes). In fact, in 1949, Moniz published a monograph, *How I Came to Perform Frontal Leucotomy*, and was awarded the Nobel Prize for Physiology or Medicine the same year.

Dr. Walter Freeman popularized the procedure and went on to develop the transorbital lobotomy, which involved using an ice-pick-like instrument called an orbitoclast. He would insert—and by insert we mean hammer—the orbitoclast through the patient's eye socket and then move it side-to-side to separate the frontal lobes from the thalamus, the part of the brain that receives and relays sensory input. However, he got carried away with doing the procedure and was eventually banned from performing it due to inappropriate use of his orbitoclast. Overall, it's estimated that about forty thousand lobotomies were done in the United States. We'll let you be the judge as to whether or not any on that list of 40K included any past elected officials.

In the 1950s, new psychotropic medications like chlorpromazine, better known as Thorazine, came out and were more effective at treating certain psychiatric conditions. That, and better long-term data showing the downside of lobotomy, helped significantly decrease the popularity of lobotomies. Public attitude toward the lobotomy also turned negative, especially after high-profile cases like that of John F. Kennedy's sister Rosemary, whose lobotomy put her in a near-vegetative state. The popular book *One Flew Over the Cuckoo's Nest*, and its movie adaptation, contributed to turning the tide of public opinion against lobotomy, too.

In hindsight, it seems clear that some of the overzealous advocates of the procedure might have benefited more from a lobotomy than their patients.

81

To Do or Not

In today's society, if two capable adults want to get married, it's nobody's business but their own. Even same-sex marriage, which, historically, has been prohibited in the United States, has now gained wide acceptance. Of course, this doesn't mean people won't give a potential bride or groom unsolicited advice. In fact, it's almost a sure thing that parents, siblings, close friends, and your weird uncle Bob all will tell you what type of guy/gal you should marry. But it's unlikely you will get such advice from your doctor in our modern times. That's what OKCupid is for!

But if we turn the clock back about ninety years, we can find some marital advice, given in full seriousness, that by modern standards seems very amusing and quaint (and quite sexist, needless to say). Take *Vitalogy: An Encyclopedia of Health and Home*, for example. The book's editor and nearly all of its authors were practicing physicians, who likely dispensed advice to their patients. Their seven rules regarding marriage are so perfectly entertaining—why not share them all here:

1. *Two people of similar complexion and temperament should never marry. If they do it will prove a failure.*
2. *Two tall, slim people or two short, heavy-set people should not marry.*
3. *A nervous, fidgety person should never marry another nervous person.*

4. A man should never marry a woman who is given to finding fault, or who is peevish and "cranky," or who scolds her little brothers and sisters.

5. A woman should never marry a man who is naturally inclined to be arrogant and cruel, or who is inordinately selfish.

6. A man should never marry a woman who is so proud that she keeps her parents poor dressing and providing for her. Beauty never atones for pride.

7. A man should never marry a woman who is "touchy" or fickle in her friendship, or often at "outs" with her parents. Depend upon it [that] these characteristics are due to a serious fault in her nature which, after marriage, will reappear in her own home to make it miserable.

And you thought Bro Code was rough.

82

Take Two Skulls and
Call Me in the Morning

The terms "medicine" and "cannibalism" are generally not used together. And that's a good thing, because the last thing U.S. health care needs is another negative association. The Commonwealth Fund rated the U.S. health care system number eleven in a 2014 review. Some might think that, all things considered, number eleven is not too bad. However, given that the Commonwealth Fund looked at eleven countries in total . . . even the basic-level mathletes see how bleak it looks. But, on the other hand, what we are about to tell you will definitely make our current health care system look great by comparison.

As reported by the German news magazine *Der Spiegel*, medical cannibalism was apparently a rather accepted practice in sixteenth- and seventeenth-century Europe. Recipes "which provided instructions on how to process human bodies, were almost as common as the use of herbs, roots and bark." The article quotes a medical historian, Richard Sugg, saying that initially powders made from shredded Egyptian mummies were used as medicine. Their popularity was based on sources like the British text *Pharmacopoeia Universalis*, which claimed that mummy flesh could cure blood clots, coughs, menstrual problems, and heal wounds.

Later, bodies of people who had been executed or "even the corpses of beggars and lepers" were utilized. The practice even spread to the British royalty. Reportedly, "Charles II paid 6,000 pounds for a recipe to distill human skull. The regent applied the resulting distillate, which entered the history of medicine as 'the king's drops,' almost daily." Those with less-kingly budgets took to standing around the scaffold with cups, hoping to catch some fresh blood as it flowed from the quivering body (it was thought to cure epilepsy). Even the moss that grows in skulls was valued, as it was thought to stop bleeding. Human fat was supposed to alleviate rheumatism and arthritis (and yet, there are some crazy people who want to give away their fat for free).

Fortunately, by the 1800s the trend of medical cannibalism was pretty much, well, consumed. We imagine that most people didn't miss the old remedies much, with the possible exception of a drink brewed by Thomas Willis, which combined powdered human skull and chocolate. Given that he must have used European chocolate, we bet even that tasted of higher quality than what gets passed off as chocolate in a certain town in Pennsylvania.

83

Itching to Add Inches

OK, we all know that penis size doesn't *really* matter, right? After all, "It's not the size of the boat but the motion of the ocean." But then again, we thought this was almost an important enough topic to deserve two entries, so . . . In fact, countless sex therapists, psychiatrists, psychologists, and others-with-no-real-expertise-except-that-they-get-to-give-advice-on-the-Internet remind us that partner satisfaction is based more on traits like honesty and open communication than size of the genitalia. This does seem to be true: based on a review of fifty studies in the *British Journal of Urology International*, 85 percent of women were satisfied with their partner's penis size.

And yet, we bet just today you've probably received a fistful (ah ha!) of e-mails advertising "safe and natural" ways to make your penis bigger (even if you are a female with no penis to start out with). Certainly, there is a cultural meme about small penises being equated with shame and inadequacy, and something that needs to be rectified by purchasing large vehicles, getting into fights, and tanning one's calves. Stand-up comedian Greg Fitzsimmons summed it up best in one line: "If you want to find guys with small penises, go to the Hummer dealership."

Given all the controversy, we didn't want to short-shrift this topic by not addressing it, so let's go deep (though not so deep as to make it painful) into the realm of all things penis. We know most of our male readers won't be able to focus on anything else until we get this out of the way: It is highly likely that your penis is not too small. As the highly respectable Mayo Clinic notes on its website, "Studies have shown that most men who think their penises are too small actually have normal-sized penises." By normal size, experts mean three to five inches of length when not erect, and five to seven inches long when erect. Anything less than three inches when erect is called a "micropenis." There. Now you can stop Googling in an incognito mode on your browser.

Back from the "bathroom break" you just had to take? (Hopefully nobody saw you take the tape measure with you.)

Good. Let's focus on those for whom having a small penis really is an issue. What can be done? If you believe that the herbal pill you just got e-mailed about actually works, you might as well also transfer some cash to the "Nigerian prince" who is waiting to send you cash. In fact, no pill or lotion has been shown to work. Vacuum pumps can make a penis larger temporarily by causing it to swell by drawing blood into it (which is how an erection usually works). However, as the Mayo Clinic points out, "Using one [a pump] too often or too long can damage elastic tissue in the penis, leading to less firm erections." How about penile exercising, aka "jelqing" or "milking," which involves pushing blood from the base to the head of the penis with one's hand? Once again, the Mayo Clinic cautions, "There's no scientific proof it works, and it can lead to scar formation, pain and disfigurement." Seriously, what did we do before the Internet?!

Unfortunately, cosmetic penis-enlargement surgery is also not a good option. At most, surgery may add half an inch to the non-erect penis, and most patients are not happy with the outcome. Potential complications can result, including the loss of sensation or function. However, there is some data (admittedly limited) that penile extenders or stretchers may be more effective (they can add half an inch or a bit more). But before you start penciling "penile extension surgery" in your calendar, know that you have to be in traction for hours every day . . . week after week . . . for many months.

So perhaps it's better to keep "willy free" and just learn to be a better rider with the motion of the ocean.

84

Pacifying Mr. Gandhi and Quieting Mister Ed

Back in the 1960s, Jack Weinberg famously said, "Don't trust anyone over thirty." Cory Doctorow revised that sentiment in 2010 in
his novel *Little Brother*, except he reduced the age to twenty-five.
Well, what would they say about an herb that has been around for
thousands of years? Some things age well with thyme. . . .

In this case, we are referring to the Indian herb sarpagandha, or
the Indian snakeroot, perhaps better known by its Latin name,
Rauvolfia serpentina, and especially known for one of its active
compounds, reserpine. Reportedly, in India this herb is part of the
traditional Ayurvedic medicine system and has been used to treat
bites from snakes (hence the Indian name) and other venomous
creatures. It has also been used in various parts of India to treat
fever, high blood pressure, insomnia, hysteria, insanity, and itching.
As reported by *Time* magazine and other sources, Alexander the
Great used this plant to cure one of his generals who had been hit
by a poisoned arrow, and Mahatma Gandhi took it as a tranquilizer
(by making tea from the dried plant).

In the West, the snakeroot was valued more for its active com-
pound reserpine, which was first isolated in 1952 from the root of
the plant and later synthesized in the lab. It has been shown to
work by blocking the uptake (and storage) of the neurotransmitters
norepinephrine and dopamine by blocking one of their transporters.

In 1979, a study published in the *Journal of the American Medical Association* demonstrated that reserpine can effectively reduce blood pressure. However, owing to its various side effects and the availability of better agents, it is rarely used now as the first-line treatment for high blood pressure. Likewise, in the 1950s reserpine was also used to treat patients with schizophrenia and other psychotic illnesses, but now it is rarely used for this purpose. Potentially dangerous side effects can include depression (although this is controversial, as some data suggests that it may actually help with depression), malignant tumors, parkinsonism, nasal congestion, and nausea.

Of note, reserpine "has been used illicitly for the sedation of show horses, for-sale horses, and in other circumstances where a 'quieter' horse might be desired." We know some people have been tempted to try this on their children, but please don't—everyone knows that children make lousy horses.

85

Everybody Gettin' Horny

When it comes to the popularity of pachyderms, rhinos do get some love in pop culture, having been featured in a range of works, from the classic literature of Rudyard Kipling's *Just So Stories* to the "hey bro" tween-culture hit *Kung Fu Panda*.

Of course, the most defining feature of the rhino is its horn. In fact, the name "rhinoceros" is derived from the Greek words *"rhin"* ("nose") and *"ceros"* ("horn"). Unfortunately, it is also the horn—or rather, human desire for it—that may lead to the extinction of this magnificent animal. Rhino horns, often shaved or ground into powder and dissolved in water or other herbal concoctions, have been traditionally used in many Asian countries for centuries. As reported by PBS's television series *Nature*, "According to the 16th century Chinese pharmacist Li Shi Chen, the horn could also cure snakebites, hallucinations, typhoid, headaches, carbuncles, vomiting, food poisoning, and 'devil possession.'" Rhino horns are highly valued in Yemen, as they are used to make handles for local daggers called *jambiya*. Fortunately, both countries banned the import of rhino horns some time ago, and for a while things were better for the rhinos.

However, a 2012 article *National Geographic* magazine stated that Vietnam has emerged as a major destination for rhino horns. Apparently, the high demand for the horns is based on rumors that a high-ranking government official successfully used rhino horn to cure his cancer. Since then, the price of rhino horn per ounce at

BENDER | KHALEGHI | SINGH

times has exceeded that of cocaine and gold. The same article reports that "Tran Quoc Binh, director of the National Hospital of Traditional Medicine, which is part of Vietnam's Ministry of Health, believe[s] that rhino horn can retard the growth of certain kinds of tumors. . . . He said that a mixture of rhino horn, ginseng, and other herbs could actually block the growth of cancer cells, but he could not produce any peer-reviewed studies to support his claims." Unfortunately, the last wild rhino in Vietnam was killed by poachers in 2010.

Although there are no credible, scientific studies that support using rhino horns for any legitimate medical purpose, we can certainly think of a part of the rhino poachers' anatomy where some might like to stick the horn.

86

Click It or Ticket!

All of us having lived in California, we grew up with the above-mentioned slogan, urging all drivers to wear their seat belts or else be ticketed. And despite all the weirdness that California is often known for, in this case it is not an outlier, as forty-nine states have laws requiring adult drivers to wear seat belts while driving (the lone exception is New Hampshire). So one would think that the fact that seat belts do indeed save lives would be incontrovertible. But, let's be honest, as a society we can't even agree on who is more an-noying, Guy Fieri with his mouth full or Paula Dean being Paula Dean, so what chance does the poor seat belt have?

Speaking for the majority opinion are institutions like the Cen-ters for Disease Control and Prevention, the National Highway Traffic Safety Administration (NHTSA), and many medical/public health organizations. The CDC, for example, clearly advocates for seat belts on its website by stating, "Adult seat belt use is the most effective way to save lives and reduce injuries in crashes" and "Seat belts reduce serious crash-related injuries and deaths by about half." The American Medical Association proudly proclaims on its website that it called for seat belts in every car as far back as 1954. And more anecdotally, almost everyone we know—Republican or Democrat—uses a seat belt and has no objection to the mandatory seat belt law.

However, there are many who question the true benefits of seat belts. An author argued in the prestigious medical journal *BMJ* that "the driving population 'risk compensated' away the substantial benefits of seatbelts by taking extra risks, putting others in more danger." That is, the author is arguing that, lulled by the sense of security and safety from seat belts, many drivers tend to drive more aggressively. The author indicates that this aggressive driving translated into greater numbers of injuries and deaths for nondrivers, like bicycle riders. An article in *Time* also claims that John Adams, a risk expert and emeritus professor of geography at University College London, has found that "mandating the use of seat belts in 18 countries resulted in either no change or actually a net increase in road accident deaths."

But before you decide to engage in conscious unbuckling, you should also know that an article by two Stanford researchers appears to split the difference. Namely, it found that seat belts do not reduce traffic fatalities as much as the NHTSA data suggest, but overall they still do reduce traffic deaths. They also did not find any substantial increased risk to nondrivers.

So we'll defer to you whether to use a seat belt or not. But at least we can all agree that texting while driving is really dangerous . . . and that Guy Fieri needs to just stop.

87

Sleep Divorce to Prevent Real Divorce?

As mundane as it may be, sleep is so important that there is a whole field of medicine dedicated to it. The number of Americans taking sleeping pills is almost as high as the number of Kanye's self-promoting tweets. (For the record, according to the Centers for Disease Control and Prevention, in 2013 about nine million Americans took prescription sleeping pills.) For better or worse, most of us who are married and light sleepers are resigned to sleeping poorly. After all, just when we have finally managed to fall asleep, our spouse happens to (inadvertently, we hope) elbow us in the face, snore louder than a lumberjack watching *Sideways*, or have an emotional emergency that requires immediate cuddling/spooning. Finally there is a solution that many are praising: sleep divorce, aka married people sleeping separately.

Although this goes against the long-established idea that married couples should share the same bed, many experts argue that data suggests sleeping alone is more beneficial. For example, Neil Stanley, a sleep researcher at the University of Surrey, reported at the British Science Festival in 2009 that, based on his research, people who shared a bed were "50 percent more likely to be disturbed during the night" than those who slept alone. As reported by the Canadian Broadcasting Company, Collen Carney, the director of Toronto's Ryerson Sleep and Depression Laboratory, found that "people will say they sleep better [together], but when we actually monitor their brains we see that their brain is not getting into deeper stages of sleep because they're continuously being woken up by movement or sound."

Lest some individuals take this as a license to make booty calls and quickly skedaddle afterward, to be fair, there is evidence arguing just the opposite. As reported in the *Wall Street Journal*, Wendy M. Troxel, an assistant professor of psychiatry and psychology at the University of Pittsburgh, found that "women in long-term stable relationships fell asleep more quickly and woke up less during the night than single women or women who lost or gained a partner during the six to eight years of the study." The article goes on to say that "one hypothesis suggests that by promoting feelings of safety and security, shared sleep in healthy relationships may lower levels of cortisol, a stress hormone. Sharing a bed may also reduce cytokines, involved in inflammation, and boost oxytocin, the so-called love hormone that is known to ease anxiety and is produced in the same part of the brain responsible for the sleep-wake cycle."

So what's the bottom line regarding the sensitive topic of sleep in marriage? We'll leave you with some words of wisdom from George Bernard Shaw: "Marriage is an alliance entered into by a man who can't sleep with the window shut, and a woman who can't sleep with the window open."

88

Doctor's Orders: Twelve Bottles of Beer, by Mouth, Daily

OK, we're talking about smallpox. But we promise the title will make sense shortly, so please read on.

Let's start with a quick primer on smallpox. The name smallpox is derived from the fifteenth-century English term "*small pockes*" ("*pocke*" meaning "sac"), although the disease is also called *variola*. But the disease is even older than its name. By some estimates, it's been around since 10,000 BC—almost as old as Kirk Douglas. References to smallpox date back two thousand to three thousand years in ancient Chinese and Indian texts. Some evidence suggests that the illness may have even later contributed to the decline of the Roman Empire. Apparently, the mummy of the Egyptian pharaoh Ramses V has lesions that resemble those of smallpox. It certainly devastated the Incan and Aztec empires after it was brought to the Americas by the conquistadores.

Smallpox was very deadly and is estimated to have killed 20 to 30 percent of infected adults, if not more. Among infants, the death rate was often as high as 80 percent. The survivors often had extensive disfiguring scars. Anything and everything was tried as a cure: herbs, cold treatments, and special cloths. In the 1600s, Thomas Sydenham, a famous English physician, apparently recommended bloodletting, emetics, travel abroad, avoiding fires, sleeping with windows opened, and "twelve Bottles of Small Beer, acidulated with Spirit of Vitriol, every Twenty Four hours."

We won't argue with those who believe that beer indeed is a miracle cure, but when it comes to smallpox, the real success came via inoculation (also called variolation). In some places, this involved introducing the powdered smallpox scabs from infected individuals into the nasal cavity of the individuals who were being inoculated. In other countries, instead of powder, pus from active smallpox lesions was taken and introduced into or under the skin of people who had not been infected. Although this was not a completely risk-free procedure—by some estimates 1 to 2 percent of individuals died—it sure was gross. Oh, and the mortality rate was about ten times lower than getting smallpox naturally.

Thankfully for those who were grossed out by the idea of having scabs and pus introduced into their bodies, Edward Jenner introduced a smallpox vaccine in 1798. The vaccine was made up of cowpox virus, which is related to the smallpox virus but causes much milder symptoms. This cowpox inoculation came to be called vaccination, and, by some estimates, Edward Jenner has saved more human lives than any other human being.

In fact, in 1979, smallpox was officially declared eradicated from the world. However, we know there are many individuals who still insist on drinking twelve bottles of beer every twenty-four hours . . . you know, just to be on the safe side.

89

Beating the Stick

It's a safe assumption that everybody knows someone who is either trying or has tried to quit smoking—and rightfully so. Consider all the dangers of smoking, including: a higher risk of getting various cancers (hence the name cancer sticks for cigarettes), heart disease, vision problems, stroke, lung disease, pneumonia, diabetes, and, for many men—a fate worse than death—erectile dysfunction. As the Centers for Disease Control and Prevention reports, smoking causes about one in five deaths in the United States and "more than 10 times as many U.S. citizens have died prematurely from cigarette smoking than have died in all the wars fought by the United States during its history."

We think most of our readers are probably also aware that some of the more common methods for smoking cessation include nicotine patches/gum/spray/lozenges, prescription medications (usually bupropion or varenicline), and therapy. Multiple studies published in prestigious journals like the *New England Journal of Medicine* do provide support for using these modalities. But there are people who would prefer to use more "natural" remedies, some of which might surprise you.

Various herbs and home remedies have been recommended as aids in smoking cessation. These include ginseng, milk thistle, St. John's Wort, red clover, licorice, valerian, honey, ginger, grapeseed extract, and many, many others. However, the data for their effectiveness is sparse, so it's difficult to recommend any of them, unless you're looking for nothing more than a good tea.

There is also anecdotal or limited evidence for other interventions. But still, some suggest that even a change in diet can help. According to F. Joseph McClernon, a researcher based at Duke University, "Loading up on fruits and vegetables even before quitting might help cigarettes seem less appealing." On the contrary, red meat, coffee, and alcohol are more likely to increase the craving for smoking. Brown University researchers have shown that vigorous exercise can almost double the quit rate. In a British study, "Smokers who cycled at a moderate pace had fewer cravings after abstaining from nicotine for 15 hours, as measured by MRI reactions to cigarette images, than non-cyclers."

Even if you are about as likely as Homer Simpson to eat right and exercise, don't worry; there is still hope. How about some advice that includes trying candy? Per Jonathan Foulds, professor of public health sciences and psychiatry at Penn State College of Medicine, "Perhaps as much as 30 percent of a smoker's cravings are actually for carbohydrates rather than nicotine." He goes on to say that the candy Jujubes reportedly has helped many people quit smoking successfully. (In the interest of full disclosure, we do not have a relationship of any kind with the company that makes Jujubes. Although we do have fond memories of eating this candy when we were children, and if the company wants to send us some free boxes, we certainly would not turn them down. Just kidding.)

Other reportedly helpful things based on some, albeit limited, data: Tai Chi, meditation, hypnosis, which may work better for men than women, acupuncture, and quitting in a group setting. Even simply talking to your doctor about smoking can be helpful. However, if you really want to be "scared straight," based on research from the University of Medicine and Dentistry of New Jersey School of Public Health, "Images of a mouth with cancerous lesions on the lips and rotten teeth, diseased lungs or a tracheotomy are potent motivators."

For a more be-kind-to-yourself approach: "In a small study at the University of Miami, researchers found that when smokers gave themselves a two-minute ear or hand massage every day for a month, they lit up less." As if men need another reason for a "hand self-massage."

90

No Wrinkle in Chyme?

The incidence of gastric (stomach) cancer in the United States is relatively low. According to the National Cancer Institute (NCI), it ranks fourteenth in incidence among the major cancers. The survival rate is rather low because the disease is usually discovered in the later stages when it has already spread. NCI estimated that in 2015 there will be 24,590 new cases of gastric cancer and 10,720 deaths. NCI lists various risk factors, including male gender, advanced age, bacterial infection with *Helicobacter pylori*, a diet high in salted, smoked, or preserved food, cigarette smoking, and various medical conditions. None of these are likely to surprise most of our readers. However, about a century ago, the list of believed risk factors included many factors that seem rather odd to us today.

According to the early-twentieth-century medical book *Vitalogy*, "a few [stomach] cancer dangers" included:

- *A broken or rough tooth causing irritation of the mouth.*
- *Eating food that is too hot or drinking liquids that scorch the esophagus or gullet.*
- *Too much sunlight in a dry, windy country where alkali dust irritates the skin.*
- *Moles or warts that stand above the surface high enough to be easily irritated.*

- *Irritation caused from the habitual smoking of a short-stem pipe.*

The implication is that by avoiding the aforementioned risk factors, one can prevent gastric cancer. However, the book is silent regarding potential treatments for this type of cancer.

Of course, the mainstream, standard treatments these days involve modalities like chemotherapy, surgery, and radiation. However, you may be surprised to learn that in a study published on August 20, 2014, in the journal *Science Translational Medicine*, the authors used Botox to slow the growth of gastric cancer in mice (and give them a youthful glow). The Botox was injected around the vagus nerve, which prevented the nerve from releasing the neurotransmitter acetylcholine. (This is the same mechanism that leads to reduced wrinkles when Botox is used for cosmetic purposes.) Acetylcholine reportedly causes cell division, so lower levels of acetylcholine subsequently result in less cell division. Furthermore, blocking acetylcholine also appeared to increase the effectiveness of the chemotherapy that the mice were also receiving. Human trials are being conducted as of this writing to determine whether Botox can be used to treat gastric cancer in the future.

And if this does pan out, perhaps finally Botox will get some respect as a legitimate medicine, and not just the favorite procedure of Hollywood celebrities and not-so-real, rich housewives.

91

Honey, I Healed the Wound!

Elsewhere in this book, we discuss the many purported uses of bee venom. We also mention that there is an entire society, the American Apitherapy Society, devoted to promoting bee products. An entire society can't survive on venom alone, so there has similarly been a lot of buzz around the beneficial effects of bee honey, allowing fans of various bee products to cross-pollinate. One of honey's sweetest features is its combination of glucose and natural fructose, which can help balance and maintain blood sugar levels during physical activity and avoid blood sugar spikes. In addition, honey's rich array of antioxidants, flavonoids, and other fancy-sounding nutrients can possibly reduce your risk of lung cancer, heart disease, Bieber Fever, and pretty much any other ailment that can give you chest pain.

Even before these long-term health benefits were discovered, honey's use in treating acute ailments had been known for thousands of years and been pretty sticky. Honey has both antifungal and antibacterial effects. In fact, honey can even fight the bacteria that most antibiotics cannot, including MRSA (methicillin-resistant *Staphylococcus aureus*). MRSA increasingly causes serious skin and hospital-acquired infections, and many consider it a major public health enemy. This makes honey, the enemy of our enemy, our friend.

Unfortunately, it's hard to consume enough honey to eradicate our internal infections, but applied topically honey may have some use. Wounds such as burns are notorious for becoming infected and so strong antibiotics are typically applied to burns while they heal. The most common of these antibiotics is silver sulfadiazine, so named because it contains both silver and sulfa, which can cause blanching of the skin, allergic reactions, and a host of other problems. Applying honey to those areas may be a healthier alternative, and this is one unusual treatment that probably actually deserves further study—we have to keep those apitherapy guys busy, after all.

Knowing these benefits, you might be tempted to spread honey on various parts of your body for medicinal or even recreational purposes. Of course, we don't judge. But please remember, while certain bugs might be repelled by honey, other bugs are quite attracted to it. So if you think you can take away that fungal jock itch by applying a little honey to the groin, you just might be trading that fungal infection for other bugs. And the last thing you want to have to tell anybody is that you are infested with bugs down there.

92

The Sad Story and Salvation of Thalidomide

When it comes to modern-day medications, there are some clear winners (Prozac) and some obvious losers (cocaine). The story of thalidomide, however, is a bit more complicated. Originally developed in the 1950s by the German company Chemie Grünenthal, it was used extensively in Europe (and later in other countries outside Europe as well) as a hypnotic (sleeping pill) and to treat morning sickness in pregnant women. It was marketed as "completely safe" and was sold as an over-the-counter drug. According to some reports, it was so popular in many countries that the amount of thalidomide used almost matched that of aspirin.

However, it did not take long for everyone to discover the terrible effects of thalidomide on the developing fetus. Many babies whose mothers had been given thalidomide as a "safe" treatment were born with severe birth defects, including phocomelia (missing or abnormal limbs, feet, or hands), missing ears, heart and kidney problems, cleft palate, spinal-cord defects, and digestive-system disorders. By 1962, thalidomide had been recalled and banned in most places. However, the maker of thalidomide, Grünenthal, refused to settle for years and blamed the birth defects on "causes like nuclear fallout or botched home abortions." It took Grünenthal fifty years to apologize to the victims of thalidomide, which finally happened in 2012.

Fortunately, in the United States, Dr. Frances Kelsey, a new hiree at the Food and Drug Administration (FDA), refused to approve thalidomide without more rigorous scientific data proving its safety. This delayed the approval long enough that likely tens of thousands of cases of severe birth defects were prevented. This also led to changes at the FDA to insure that all future approved medications would have to meet a higher standard for safety.

However, in a rather ironic twist, thalidomide's propensity to restrict blood-vessel growth (which resulted in phocomelia) also makes it useful in treating certain medical conditions, such as some cancerous tumors, multiple myeloma, Crohn's disease, and multiple sclerosis. In Brazil it has been used for some time now to treat leprosy as well. (The FDA approved thalidomide for leprosy in 1998.) Unfortunately, although there are more safeguards now regarding the usage of thalidomide, especially in pregnant women, approximately one hundred children with thalidomide-induced disabilities have been born in Brazil since 2005. Hopefully with additional education and possible safeguards, the number can be reduced to zero.

93

Finding *Frankenstein's* Fountainhead

Most people have heard about the fictional monster created by Dr. Frankenstein, even if they have not read the original book of the same name or gone on a match.com date. *Frankenstein* was published anonymously by Mary Shelley in 1818 and considered one of the first science-fiction books ever written. There are many who postulate that there are some interesting potential connections between the idea of Frankenstein's monster and medicine and physicians of that era.

As reported by *Time*, Mary Shelley, in a preface to her novel, claimed to have been inspired by a nightmare she had while staying in Geneva with Percy Shelley and Lord Byron. However, even as a child, whether consciously or not, Mary was likely influenced by other sources with close ties to medicine. For instance, Erasmus Darwin, the grandfather of Charles Darwin and a physician, was a good friend of Mary's father and very interested in the idea of galvanism, the contraction of muscles when stimulated with electricity. Mary mentions this in her preface as well. As reported by *Mental Floss*, Giovanni Aldini, in 1803, "staged a public demonstration of galvanism at the Royal College of Surgeons in London using the body of murderer George Forster shortly after he was executed. He was able to make the corpse's face grimace and the arms and legs to flex violently by applying electrodes connected to a battery."

(*NSYNC was paid to dance like this all on their own.) This scene is thought to have been witnessed by a family friend of Mary Shelley's household and reported in detail to her father (and overheard by Mary).

A more personal connection may have been Henry Cline, who had been Mary Shelley's doctor at one time. Dr. Cline was a local celebrity for having revived a sailor who had been comatose for months. A friend of Mary's husband, Dr. James Lind, experimented with animal electricity, and reportedly applied electricity to frog legs to make them move.

While none of these "prove" a direct connection between Mary Shelley's idea and the idea of reanimation or bringing the dead back to life prevalent in medicine of that era, it's quite plausible that the accumulation of such beliefs influenced Mary Shelley. The other monster-related mystery we would love to answer is what inspired Bobby Pickett's "Monster Mash." A bad batch of LSD, binging on fructose-corn-syruped candy, and watching *House of Dracula* too many times?

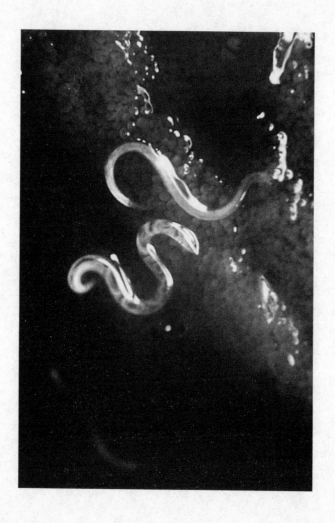

A photo of worms, providing helminthic therapy.
Credit: The Centers for Disease Control and Prevention. Public Domain.

94

Guess I'll Go Eat Worms

Let's face it, worms get no respect in our culture. Say the word "worm" to someone, and most likely, the next word to pop up in the head is "lowly." Not to mention all the people who have been traumatized upon biting into an apple and discovering the wiggling remnant of a half-eaten wiggler—an experience only slightly less gross than eating three Taco Bell chalupas back to back. Or so we've heard. But there is nothing Americans love more than the stories of underdogs making it big . . . and in that sense, the worm has turned for the worm and it is starting to play an important role in medicine.

Helminthic therapy is the fancy name for using certain worms (helminths, like hookworm and whipworm) to treat various autoimmune disorders, such as multiple sclerosis, Crohn's disease, ulcerative colitis, and inflammatory bowel disease. Although the full explanation of why this therapy works has not been elucidated, many experts in this field believe that it relates to the hygiene hypothesis. The idea behind this hypothesis is that historically certain infectious agents and parasites infected humans, which is no longer the case owing to changes in our environment. Although this has resulted in our reduced exposure to some dangerous organisms— clearly a good thing—it has also contributed to fewer infections with benign, and possibly even beneficial, organisms. Without the experiences of these infections, our immune system's development is altered, making us more susceptible to various autoimmune disorders.

This idea is further supported by the fact that in certain developing countries in sub-Saharan Africa and Asia, where parasitic infections are more common, the rates of autoimmune disorders are significantly lower.

As to how helminthic therapy works, the details are still unclear. But it seems that infection with helminths results in the suppression of certain inflammatory immune molecules and higher levels of other benign molecules. For example, a man featured in a *Scientific American* article swallowed "a vial of salty liquid brimming with 500 human whipworm eggs" in an effort to treat his ulcerative colitis, followed by another ingestion. After a few months, he was "virtually symptom free." He relapsed later when the number of eggs in his body decreased, but he again responded well to further ingestions. Researchers discovered that when his illness was more active, his immune cells produced large quantities of an immune molecule called interleukin-17 (IL-17), which causes inflammation. At the same time, he had low levels of interleukin-22 (IL-22), which is associated with wound healing and mucus production. When worms were reintroduced to his gut, the levels of IL-22 increased and he felt better.

Although these worms may be redeeming themselves, there is simply no excuse for earworms like "It's a Small World." It definitely increases our inflammatory bowel response.

95

One of the Few Practices
We Endorse

OK, we don't really endorse anything unsafe. Fortunately, many of the "natural" ways to make your breasts bigger are perfectly safe and even healthy. You can do exercises that build your chest muscles, such as push-ups and chest flies, which technically just push up the breasts, but we don't think most people care about this distinction. You can also eat lots of healthy protein and fats to support tissue formation, although eating too much may counter the desired results. Where we draw the line is anything unstudied, unproven, or with any health risks no matter what the alleged benefit is to women . . . and, indirectly, some men.

Increasing estrogen can increase breast size, but estrogen supplements have been associated with health risks such as blood clots and certain reproductive cancers, which is not the way breasts should be made bigger. A safer plan may be to eat foods that naturally increase your own production of estrogen, or phytoestrogens such as flax seeds and soy, which have plenty of other health benefits as well. Even in men there is concern that these foods can increase estrogen and contribute to gynecomastia, the fancy medical term for man boobs.

Many herbs have been suggested for breast enlargement, including fenugreek, saw palmetto, and wild yam. We are less fans of herbs than of food because there is less evidence and research that support the use of high-dose herbs. Many people feel herbs are safe because they are "natural," but so are strychnine and cyanide.

For those women who feel the need to enlarge their breasts to appear more appealing to men, studies show that many men do not necessarily find larger breasts more attractive. In fact, more intelligent men are often more attracted to eyes or legs, since they reveal facets of personality and athleticism, respectively. Only men who are boobs just look at . . . well . . . boobs.

96

Getting Pissy

There's no use in denying it: this has been a bad week.
I've started drinking my own urine.

—AMERICAN PSYCHO by Bret Easton Ellis

Drinking urine is not an activity limited to fictional characters. This practice, which has followers all over the world, often goes by the more fancy-sounding name "urotherapy." However, that name does absolutely nothing to make it any more palatable.

According to one highly skeptical reference, the conditions that urotherapy supposedly help include: cold and flu, broken bones, toothaches, skin conditions, asthma, heart disease, obesity, hypertension, burns, cancer, poison, animal bites, constipation, dysentery, and gastric ulcers . . . and the list goes on and on, as do many completely made-up lists of cure-alls.

Although the medical establishment in general does not support any of these claims, the BBC did report that at least one physician was "instructing patients to collect their own urine in the morning and drink it untreated, starting with small amounts and progressing to a glassful a day." Question: What do you think *that* doctor's been drinking?

Consider this more "sophisticated" approach to drinking only the finest urine, based on a real-life medical encounter:

A forty-year-old man presented to the emergency room with complaints of pain when urinating. He reported no unprotected sex, no discharge from his penis, and no recent injuries to his genitals. His urine sample showed the presence of bacteria in the patient's urine and a urinary tract infection (UTI). In younger, healthy men, UTIs are uncommon and are typically caused by unusual anatomy. For that reason, the ER doctor ordered an X-ray of the patient's kidneys, ureter, and bladder. Result: normal.

After the doctor told the patient of the UTI, the patient said, "I should have known. This does happen to me every now and then, usually after work." The patient explained, "I'm a human decanter. I get hired by people to serve wine at their parties."

The doctor was puzzled—until the patient elaborated.

"I think it has to do with how I serve the wine. . . . See, I get a catheter and insert it into my penis. I pour in a bottle of wine or two, and then I pee the wine out into glasses."

"And the people who hire you know that you do this?" asked the startled doctor.

"Of course!" the patient answered, offended. "What kind of a sick person do you think I am?"

What wine bouquet do you think the sommelier picked up in those glasses?

References

1. The Creepiest of All Treatments
Carrie Arnold, "New Science Shows How Maggots Heal Wounds," accessed December 20, 2014, www.scientificamerican.com/article/news-science-shows-how-maggots-heal-wounds.
Paul Gabrielsen, "How Maggots Heal Wounds," accessed December 17, 2014, news .sciencemag.org/2012/12/how-maggots-heal-wounds.

2. More Doctors Smoke Camels . . . Well, What Else Would You Do to a Camel?
Martha N. Gardner and Allan M. Brandt, "'The Doctors' Choice Is America's Choice': The Physician in U.S. Cigarette Advertisements, 1930–1953," *American Journal of Public Health* 96 (2006): 222–32, accessed April 21, 2015, www.ncbi.nlm.nih.gov/pmc/articles /PMC1470496/pdf/0960222.pdf.
Hadgirl, "10 Evil Vintage Cigarette Ads Promising Better Health," accessed April 21, 2015, www .healthcare-administration-degree.net/10-evil-vintage-cigarette-ads-promising-better-health.
"Your Doctor Wants You to Smoke," accessed April 21, 2015, content.time.com/time /photogallery/0,29307,1848212,00.html.

3. Stuck on You
David Kim, e-mail message to author, October 2, 2015.

4. Want Fries with That?
"Bleed-X: Vet Hemostatic Powder," accessed June 13, 2015, www.dvmsolutions.com /bleed-x.htm.
Gurkan Ersoy et al., "Hemostatic Effects of Microporous Polysaccharide Hemosphere in a Rat Model with Severe Femoral Artery Bleeding," *Advances in Therapy* (Impact Factor: 2.44) 24 (2007): 485–92, accessed June 13, 2015, doi:10.1007/BF02848770.
Sara Israels, Nora Schwetz, Ron Boyar, and Archie McNicol, "Bleeding Disorders: Characterization, Dental Considerations and Management," *Journal of the Canadian Dental Association* 72 (2006): 827–827l, accessed July 11, 2015, umanitoba.ca/health -sciences/dentistry/media/IsraelsJCDA.pdf.

5. Unwrinkling a Wizard's Sleeve?

"Botox Injection for Treatment of Vaginismus," accessed June 13, 2015, clinicaltrials.gov/ct2/show/NCT01352546.

"Frequently Asked Questions (FAQs) about Infant Botulism," accessed July 12, 2015, www.infantbotulism.org/general/faq.php.

"Vaginismus," accessed June 13, 2015, www.vaginismusmd.com.

6. Placenta: It's Not Just for Breakfast Anymore

Laura Devlin, "Why Do People Eat Placentas?," accessed December 26, 2014, www.bbc.com/news/uk-england-27307476.

"Insufficient Evidence to Support Health Claims Associated with Eating Placenta," accessed December 26, 2014, africacheck.org/reports/insufficient-evidence-to-support-health-claims-associated-with-eating-placenta/#sthash.oaUF6xTN.dpuf.

Kimberly Leonard, "Moms: Should You Eat Your Placenta?," US News, May 9, 2014, accessed December 26, 2014, health.usnews.com/health-news/health-wellness/articles/2014/05/09/moms-should-you-eat-your-placenta.

7. Does This Jersey Make Me Look Fat?

Pierre Chandon, "Backing the Wrong Sports Team Can Make You Fat," Forbes, August 28, 2013, accessed December 27, 2014, www.forbes.com/sites/insead/2013/08/28/backing-the-wrong-sports-team-can-make-you-fat.

Jan Hoffman, "When Teams Lose, Fans Tackle Fatty Foods," New York Times, September 16, 2013, accessed December 27, 2014, well.blogs.nytimes.com/2013/09/16/when-teams-lose-fans-tackle-fatty-food.

Nick McDermott, "How a Bad Football Team Makes You Fat: Supporting the Losing Team Causes Fans to Binge on Fatty, Sugar-Laden Food Following a Defeat," Daily Mail, August 21, 2013, last modified August 22, 2013, accessed December 27, 2014, www.dailymail.co.uk/health/article-2398790/Supporting-losing-football-team-causes-fans-binge-following-defeat.html#ixzz3N7SG1FST.

8. A Sting to Treat a Sting

"Apitherapy: Homeopathic Bee Venom Therapy," accessed January 10, 2015, www.holisticmd.org/treatments/apitherapy-homeopathic-bee-venom-therapy.

"Study Shows that Bee Venom Can Kill Hepatitis B, C, and Cancer Cells," accessed January 9, 2015, www.datalounge.com/cgi-bin/iowa/ajax.html?t=12560988#page:showThread,12560988.

9. You Can't Redo Everything

Robert B. Bluey, "Congresswoman Wants 'Rebirthing' Therapy Outlawed," accessed December 29, 2014, cnsnews.com/news/article/congresswoman-wants-rebirthing-therapy-outlawed.

Julie Cart, "2 Convicted in Girl's Death During 'Rebirthing' Therapy," Los Angeles Times,

April 21, 2001, accessed December 29, 2014, articles.latimes.com/2001/apr/21/news
/mn-53812.

"Just What Is Rebirthing Therapy?," accessed December 19, 2014, www.webmd.com/mental
-health/news/20000628/rebirthing-therapy.

"'Rebirthing' Therapist Denies Guilt," accessed December 29, 2014, abcnews.go.com/2020
/story?id=124076.

10. Country Music Can Be Deadly (for White People)

Aishwarya, "There Is a Positive Correlation between Country Music and Suicide Rates in
Metropolitan Areas," accessed December 29, 2014, www.omgfacts.com/lists/10984/There-is
-a-positive-correlation-between-country-music-and-suicide-rates-in-metropolitan-areas.

Mark James Shultz, "Don't Let Your Sons Grow Up to be Cowboys: Country Music Causes
Suicide?!," accessed December 29, 2014, www.personal.psu.edu/afr3/blogs/siowfa13/2013
/10/dont-let-your-sons-grow-up-to-be-cowboys-country-music-causes-suicide.html.

Steven Stack and Jim Gundlach, "The Effect of Country Music on Suicide," *Social Forces* 71,
no. 1 (1992): 211–18, accessed December 29, 2014, comp.uark.edu/~ches/CountryMusic
_Suicide.pdf.

11. Dark Days: Experimentation on Mentally Challenged and Mentally Ill Patients

Institutional Review Board Guidebook, Chapter VI: Special Classes of Subjects, last modified
1993, accessed December 30, 2014, www.hhs.gov/ohrp/archive/irb/irb_chapter6.htm.

Lauren Davis, "Six Abandoned Asylums with Genuinely Chilling Backstories," accessed
December 30, 2014, io9.com/six-abandoned-asylums-with-genuinely-chilling-backstori
-512154481.

"Fernald State School," accessed December 30, 2014, www.asylumprojects.org/index.php
?title=Fernald_State_School.

Olga Khazan, "Pulling Teeth to Treat Mental Illness," *Atlantic,* October 22, 2014, accessed
December 30, 2014, www.theatlantic.com/health/archive/2014/10/the-tragic-sadistic
-mental-illness-treatment-from-the-knick-is-real/381751.

Boston Globe, "Quaker Oats, MIT to Pay $1.85 Million: Mass. Residents Were Fed
Radiation-Spiked Cereal," *Baltimore Sun,* December 31, 1997, accessed December 30,
2014, articles.baltimoresun.com/1997-12-31/news/1997365029_1_quaker-oats-mit
-researchers.

"Trenton State Hospital," accessed December 30, 2014, www.asylumprojects.org/index.php
?title=Trenton_State_Hospital.

12. Stretch Armstrong's Got Nothing on This!

B. Vargas Bareto et al., "Complications of Ilizarov Leg Lengthening: A Comparative
Study between Patients with Leg Length Discrepancy and Short Stature," *International
Orthopaedics* 31 (2007): 587–91, accessed January 1, 2015, doi:10.1007/s00264-006
-0236-2.

"Distraction Osteogenesis," accessed January 1, 2015, www.seattlechildrens.org/clinics
-programs/craniofacial/services/distraction.

"Distraction Osteogenesis," accessed January 1, 2015, en.wikipedia.org/wiki/Distraction
_osteogenesis.

B. Spiegelberg et al., "Ilizarov Principles of Deformity Correction," *Annals of the Royal College
of Surgeons of England* 92 (2010): 101–5, accessed January 1, 2015, doi:10.1308/0035884
10X12518836439326.

Peter van Strijen et al., "Complications in Bilateral Mandibular Distraction Osteogenesis," *Oral
Surgery, Oral Medicine, Oral Pathology, and Oral Radiology* 96 (2003): 392–97, accessed
January 1, 2015, doi:10.1016/S1079-2104(03)00472-4.

"The Use of the Ilizarov Method in Children for Limb Lengthening," accessed January 1, 2015,
www.medscape.com/viewarticle/722302_2.

13. Two Eyes, Two Ears, Two Noses?

Tia Ghose, "Man's 'Forehead Nose' a Common Reconstruction Technique," accessed January
3, 2015, www.livescience.com/39942-forehead-nose-normal-procedure.html.

Donald M. Greer, Jr., Paul C. Mohl, and Kathy A. Sheley, "A Technique for Foreskin Reconstruction and Some Preliminary Results," *Journal of Sex Research* 18, no. 4 (1982): 324–30,
accessed January 3, 2015, www.cirp.org/library/restoration/greer1.

Gillian Mohney, "Doctors Grow Nose on Man's Forehead," accessed January 3, 2015, abcnews
.go.com/blogs/health/2013/09/25/doctors-grow-nose-on-mans-forehead.

Chris O'Neill, "How and Why to Regrow Your Foreskin," accessed January 3, 2015,
www.vice.com/en_uk/read/how-and-why-to-regrow-your-foreskin.

"Tissue Expansion," accessed January 3, 2015, en.wikipedia.org/wiki/Tissue_expansion.

"Xiaolian, Chinese Man, Grows New Nose on Forehead," accessed January 3, 2015,
www.huffingtonpost.co.uk/2013/09/25/china-man-nose-forehead_n_3988678
.html?utm_hp_ref=uk.

14. I Need This Like I Need a Hole in the Head!

Will Stewart and Jonathan O'Callaghan, "Brain Surgery, the Ancient Way: Scientists Try Out
2,500-Year-Old Method Used to Treat Epilepsy and Headaches on a Modern Skull," *Daily
Mail*, January 30, 2015, accessed February 4, 2015, www.dailymail.co.uk/sciencetech/article
-2932940/Brain-surgery-ANCIENT-way-Scientists-try-2-500-year-old-method-used-treat
-epilepsy-headaches-modern-skull.html.

Allan Tasman, Jerald Kay, et al., *Psychiatry*, 3rd ed., vol. 1 (Hoboken, NJ: Wiley, 2008).

"Trepanning in Prehistoric Times," *New York Times,* February 4, 1883, accessed February 1,
2015, timesmachine.nytimes.com/timesmachine/1883/02/04/102808519.html
?pageNumber=4.

"Trepanning," accessed February 1, 2015, en.wikipedia.org/wiki/Trepanning.

Christopher Turner, "Like a Hole in the Head," *Cabinet,* Winter 2007/2008, accessed February
4, 2015, cabinetmagazine.org/issues/28/turner.php.

REFERENCES

15. Asthma, Allergies, and Long-Term Worms

"Evidence for the Use of the Immunotherapy Helminthic Therapy to Treat Anaphylaxis and Peanut Allergy," accessed March 15, 2015, autoimmunetherapies.com/candidate _diseases_for_helminthic_therapy_or_worm_therapy/peanut_allergies_anaphylaxis .html.

Robbie Gonzalez, "Why Doctors Are Treating Allergies with Parasitic Worms," accessed March 15, 2015, io9.com/5933615/why-doctors-are-treating-allergies-with-parasitic -worms.

"Hookworms and Allergies—Doctor Infects Himself for Experiment," accessed March 10, 2015, www.medicalnewstoday.com/articles/244238.php.

R. J. Quinnell, J. Bethony, and D. I. Pritchard, "The Immunoepidemiology of Human Hookworm Infection," *Parasite Immunology* 26 (2004): 443–54, accessed March 15, 2015, doi:10.1111/j.0141-9838.2004.00727.x.

Elizabeth Svoboda, "Can Hookworms Protect Against Allergies?," *New York Times,* July 1, 2008, accessed March 15, 2015, www.nytimes.com/2008/07/01/health/01iht-01prof .14122951.html?_r=0.

16. The G-Spot Shot: Spot On or Spot Off?

Ernst Gräfenberg, "The Role of Urethra in Female Orgasm," *International Journal of Sexology* 3 (1950): 145–48, accessed March 25, 2015, www.landman-psychology.com/284/sexuality /grafenberg-gspot.htm.

"G-Shot for Your G-Spot: Vagina Injection Said to Enhance Sexual Pleasure Gains Popularity," accessed March 24, 2015, www.huffingtonpost.com/2012/10/23/g-shot-g-spot-vagina -injection-enhance-sexual-pleasure_n_2005732.html.

Vincenzo Puppo and Ilan Gruenwald, "Does the G-spot Exist? A Review of the Current Literature," *International Urogynecology Journal* 23 (2012): 1665–69, accessed March 24, 2015, doi:10.1007/s00192-012-1831-y.

17. Chakra the Monkey Tonight!

"Chakra," accessed April 6, 2015, en.wikipedia.org/wiki/Chakra.

Michelle Fondin, "What Is a Chakra?," accessed April 7, 2015, www.chopra.com/ccl/what-is-a -chakra.

Zain Saraswati Jamal, "Balance Your Chakras with Food," accessed April 10, 2015, www .gaiamtv.com/article/balance-your-chakras-food.

Reshma Patel, "Warning Signs Your Chakras Are Out of Balance," accessed April 10, 2015, www.mindbodygreen.com/0-13433/warning-signs-your-chakras-are-out-of-balance.html.

"Reiki Healing Health Benefits," accessed April 10, 2015, www.reiki-for-holistic-health.com/.

18. Moxibustion: Not Quite Smoking Banana Leaves, but Almost!

"Acupuncture Points and Meridians," accessed April 12, 2015, www.acupuncture-meridians .com/#Acupoints_meridians.

REFERENCES

Myeong Soo Lee et al., "Moxibustion for Cancer Care: A Systematic Review and Meta-analysis," *BMC Cancer* 10 (2010): 1–8, accessed April 13, 2015, doi:10.1186/1471-2407-10.

"Moxibustion," accessed April 10, 2015 (no longer available), www.cancer.org/treatment /treatmentsandsideeffects/complementaryandalternativemedicine/manualhealingand physicaltouch/moxibustion.

"Moxibustion," accessed April 10, 2015, en.wikipedia.org/wiki/Moxibustion#cite_note-acs-1.

"Treating Face Paralysis by Traditional Chinese Medicine," accessed April 10, 2015 (no longer available), chinesemedicinenews.com/2007/06/15/treating-face-paralysis-by-traditional -chinese-medicine-photo-story.

19. Maybe They Just Passed Gas

Jim H., "The 21 Grams Theory," accessed April 14, 2015, www.historicmysteries.com/the-21 -gram-soul-theory.

Benjamin Radford, "How Much Does the Soul Weigh?," accessed April 14, 2015, www .livescience.com/32327-how-much-does-the-soul-weigh.html.

"Soul Has Weight, Physician Thinks," *New York Times,* March 11, 1907, accessed April 14, 2015, query.nytimes.com/mem/archive-free/pdf?res=9D07E5DC123EE033A25752C1A965 9C946697D6CF.

"Soul Man," accessed July 12, 2015, www.snopes.com/religion/soulweight.asp.

20. As If Birth Weren't Traumatic Enough

"The Basics of Water Birth," www.waterbirth.com. Accessed October 20, 2014.

"Immersion in Water During Labor and Delivery," accessed April 21, 2015, www.acog.org /Resources-And-Publications/Committee-Opinions/Committee-on-Obstetric-Practice /Immersion-in-Water-During-Labor-and-Delivery.

"Water Birth: The Benefits and Risks," accessed April 21, 2015, americanpregnancy.org/labor -and-birth/water-birth.

"Waterbirth International," accessed April 21, 2015, www.waterbirth.org.

21. An Eerie Enema

Siu Fai Lo et al., "Traumatic Rectal Perforation by an Eel," *Surgery* 135 (2004): 110–11, accessed February 22, 2015, doi:10.1016/S0039-6060(03)00076-X.

www.mucusfreelife.com/ehret-library/overview/arnold-ehret/tragedy-of-nutrition. Accessed November 2, 2014.

Katsumi Tsukamoto and Mari Kuroki, eds., *Eels and Humans* (New York: Springer, 2014), 58–59.

22. They Say Stripes Are Slimming

"Arsenic Early in Treatment Improves Survival for Leukemia Patients," accessed April 21, 2015, www.wakehealth.edu/News-Releases/2010/Arsenic_Early_in_Treatment_Improves _Survival_for_Leukemia_Patients.htm.

"Bronze, Humbugs, Wallpaper and Electronics: What's Your Favourite Element?," accessed April 21, 2015, thechronicleflask.wordpress.com/tag/bradford-sweets-poisoning.

Esther Inglis-Arkell, "Arsenic Poisoning May Have Spawned Two Different Movie Monsters," accessed April 21, 2015, io9.com/arsenic-poisoning-may-have-spawned-two-different -movie-672335981.

Steven Marcus, "Arsenic Toxicity," accessed April 21, 2015, emedicine.medscape.com/article /812953-overview.

23. Ping-Pong, Anyone?

"Older Methods of Treating TB, Plombage Therapy, 'Ping-Pong Ball Plombage,'" accessed April 22, 2015, www.learningradiology.com/archives03/COW%20049-Ping%20Pong%20 Plumbage/plombagecorrect.htm.

Stéphane Jouveshomme et al., "Preliminary Results of Collapse Therapy with Plombage for Pulmonary Disease Caused by Multidrug-Resistant Mycobacteria," *American Journal of Respiratory and Critical Care Medicine* 157 (1998): 1609–15, accessed April 22, 2015, doi:10.1164/ajrccm.157.5.9709047.

Sumit Yadav, Hemant Sharma, and Anand Iyer, "Late Extrusion of Pulmonary Plombage Outside the Thoracic Cavity," *Interactive Cardiovascular and Thoracic Surgery* 10 (2010): 808–10, accessed April 22, 2015, doi:10.1510/icvts.2009.22069.

"Tuberculosis," accessed April 22, 2015, www.cdc.gov/tb.

"What Is Plombage?," accessed April 22, 2015, www.wisegeek.com/what-is-plombage .htm.

24. Treating Hemorrhoids: A Real Pain in the Butt

"Hemorrhoids: Causes, Symptoms, and Treatments," accessed April 22, 2015, www .medicalnewstoday.com/articles/73938.php.

"How Hemorrhoids Were Treated in Historical Times," accessed April 22, 2015, weird-diseases .blogspot.com/2014/06/how-hemorrhoids-were-treated-in.html.

David Morton, "10 Excruciating Medical Treatments from the Middle Ages," accessed April 22, 2015, www.oddee.com/item_96620.aspx.

"St. Fiacre? Patron Saint of Hemorrhoid Sufferers," accessed April 22, 2015, wellvillesite .squarespace.com/culture/2011/1/10/st-fiacre-patron-saint-of-hemorrhoid-sufferers.html.

25. Sore Throat: Better or Worse After These Remedies?

W. E. Baldwin, *Essential Lessons in Human Physiology and Hygiene for Schools* (New York; Chicago; Boston: Werner School Book Company, 1898), 171.

Amie M. Hale and T. E. C., Jr., "The Value of a Salt Pork Compress in the Treatment of a Child with Sore Throat," *Pediatrics* 63 (1979): 527, accessed April 22, 2015, pediatrics .aappublications.org/content/63/4/527.

Wayland D. Hand, *Magical Medicine: The Folkloric Component of Medicine in the Folk*

Belief, Custom, and Ritual of the Peoples of Europe and America: Selected Essays of Wayland D. Hand (Berkeley; Los Angeles; London: University of California Press, 1980), 326.

Elisabeth Janos, *Country Folk Medicine: Tales of Skunk Oil, Sassafras Tea, and Other Old-Time Remedies* (New York: Galahad Books, 1995): 80–81.

26. Facing the Facts When, in Fact, That's Not Your Face

Naomi Austin, " 'My Face Transplant Saved Me,' " accessed April 23, 2015, news.bbc.co.uk/2 /hi/health/6058696.stm.

"Amazing Face Transplants (Graphic Images)," accessed April 23, 2015, www.cbsnews.com /pictures/amazing-face-transplants-graphic-images.

"Face Transplant," accessed April 23, 2015, www.brighamandwomens.org/About_BWH /publicaffairs/news/facetransplant/default.aspx?sub=0.

"Saving Face: Spanish Hospital Performs World's Most Complex 'Face Transplant,' " accessed April 23, 2015, rt.com/news/245481-spain-face-transplant-hospital.

"University of Maryland Completes Most Comprehensive Face Transplant Performed to Date," accessed April 23, 2015, umm.edu/programs/face-transplant/media-resources.

27. Stocks Drop, So Might the Bodies

Joseph Engelberg and Christopher A. Parsons, "Worrying about the Stock Market: Evidence from Hospital Admissions," accessed April 23, 2015, rady.ucsd.edu/faculty/directory /engelberg/pub/portfolios/HEALTH.pdf.

Alan Farnham, "When Stocks Drop, Heart Attacks Rise," accessed April 23, 2015, abcnews.go .com/Business/stocks-decline-heart-attacks-increase/story?id=21434968.

Mona Fiuzat et al., "United States Stock Market Performance and Acute Myocardial Infarction Rates in 2008–2009 (from the Duke Databank for Cardiovascular Disease)," *American Journal of Cardiology* 106 (2010): 1545–49, accessed April 23, 2015, doi:10.1016/j .amjcard.2010.07.027.

Bryan Glen Schwartz et al., "How the 2008 Stock Market Crash and Seasons Affect Total and Cardiac Deaths in Los Angeles County," *American Journal of Cardiology* 109 (2012): 1445–48, accessed April 23, 2015, doi:10.1016/j.amjcard.2012.01.354.

Chris Wang, "Is the Stock Market Going to Kill You?," accessed April 23, 2015, www .huffingtonpost.com/chris-wang/is-the-stock-recession-depression_b_4665600.html.

28. It's Just a Flesh Wound

Barry Eppley, "Plastic Surgery History: Burn Surgery and the Walking Tubed Pedicle Flap," accessed April 23, 2015, www.exploreplasticsurgery.com/tag/tubed-pedicle-flap.

"In Pictures: Faces of Battle," accessed April 23, 2015, news.bbc.co.uk/2/shared/spl/hi/picture _gallery/07/magazine_faces_of_battle/html/6.stm.

Grace Murano, "World's First Plastic Surgeries," accessed April 23, 2015, www.oddee.com/item _98767.aspx.

Maurice Y. Nahabedian, "Free Tissue Transfer Flaps," accessed April 23, 2015, emedicine
.medscape.com/article/1284841-overview.

29. When Blood Is Green and Urine Blue

Alana M. Flexman, Giuseppe Del Vicario, and Stephan K. W. Schwarz, "Dark Green Blood in
the Operating Theatre," *Lancet* 369 (2007): 1972, accessed April 23, 2015, doi:10.1016
/S0140-6736(07)60918-0.

"Man Oozes Green Blood Before Operation," accessed April 23, 2015, www.foxnews.com
/story/2007/06/11/man-oozes-green-blood-before-operation.

Becky Oskin, "Pee a Rainbow: Scientist Snaps Shot of Colorful Urine," accessed April 23, 2015,
www.livescience.com/37664-human-urine-colors-rainbow.html.

"Patient Bleeds Dark Green Blood," accessed April 23, 2015, news.bbc.co.uk/2/hi/health
/6733203.stm.

30. Prosthetic Limbs of Today: Beyond Pegs and Hooks

Isha Aran, "Cops Arrest Woman After Drugs Fall Out of Her Prosthetic Butt," accessed
April 25, 2015, jezebel.com/cops-arrest-woman-after-drugs-fall-out-of-her-prostheti
-1642502728.

Sarah Fecht, "Feedback System Lets Amputees 'Feel' Prosthetic Leg," accessed April 25, 2015,
www.popularmechanics.com/science/health/a12060/feedback-system-lets-amputees-feel
-prosthetic-leg-14821609.

Barbara Hijek, "Report: Deputies Found Drugs in Prosthetic Leg, Bra; Needle Hidden in Woman's
Butt during Traffic Stop," accessed April 25, 2015, articles.sun-sentinel.com/2013-03-01/news
/sfl-prosthetic-leg-woman-needle-butt-20130228_1_prosthetic-leg-deputies-needle.

S. Uchida et al., "Side-Effects of Prosthetic Materials on the Human Body," *International
Orthopaedics* 3 (1980): 285–91, accessed April 25, 2015, link.springer.com/article/10.1007
/BF00266023.

31. Want Bigger Breasts? Have a Thai Stranger Slap Them Repeatedly

Joseph Bien-Kahn, "For $350, Tata Will Slap You Until You're Sexy," accessed April 26, 2015,
www.vice.com/read/for-350-tata-will-slap-your-face-until-your-pretty.

"Breast Slapping—A Natural Alternative to Plastic Surgery," accessed April 26, 2015, www
.growbreastsnaturally.com/breast-slapping-a-natural-alternative-to-plastic-surgery.html.

Daisy Dumas, "Nothing Like a Bit of Slap: Bizarre Thai Beauty Treatment Sees Therapist Hit
Breasts to Make Them Larger," accessed April 26, 2015, www.dailymail.co.uk/femail/article
-2039764/Thai-breast-slapping-therapist-claims-hitting-boobs-makes-bigger.html.

32. Truly Giving a Shit

"BART Escalators: Poop Responsible For Breaking Feces-Clogged Equipment," accessed
June 13, 2015, www.huffingtonpost.com/2012/07/26/broken-bart-escalators-poop_n
_1706716.html.

"Fecal Matter Found on 72 Percent of Grocery Carts," accessed June 13, 2015, www.foxnews
.com/health/2011/03/03/fecal-matter-72-percent-grocery-carts.

"Fecal transplants dramatically improve C. difficile in kids" accessed November 5, 2015, www
.mayoclinic.org/medical-professionals/clinical-updates/digestive-diseases/fecal-transplants
-dramatically-improve-c-diff-in-kids.

33. "Hands-On" Help for Hysteria

Michael Castleman, "Hysteria and the Strange History of Vibrators," accessed June 14, 2015,
www.psychologytoday.com/blog/all-about-sex/201303/hysteria-and-the-strange-history
-vibrators.

34. Kim Kardashian's Vampire Facial (No, Not *That* Kind!)

Ruthie Friedlander, "I Got the Kim Kardashian Vampire Facial," accessed June 14, 2015,
www.elle.com/beauty/makeup-skin-care/news/a14931/kim-kardashians-vampire-facial.

Richard M. Goldfarb and Aaron L. Shapiro, "Benefits of Autologous Fat Grafting Using
Fat Mixed with Platelet-Rich Fibrin Matrix (PRFM) Selphyl," *American Journal of Cosmetic
Surgery* 29 (2012): 62–64, accessed June 14, 2015, doi:10.5992/AJCS-D-11-00037.1.

Mia Taylor, "$1500 Buys a Kim Kardashian Vampire Facial," accessed June 14, 2015, www
.thestreet.com/story/12712922/1/1500-buys-a-kim-kardashian-vampire-facial.html.

35. MADW Wasn't Quite as Catchy

Diana Huynh, "The Perils of Drunk Walking," accessed September 14, 2014, freakonomics.com
/2011/12/28/the-perils-of-drunk-walking.

36. A Load of Bully

Gwen Dewar, "The Road to Psychopathy: Why Bullying in Children Affects Us All," accessed
October 12, 2014, www.parentingscience.com/bullying-in-children.html.

37. Why Didn't They Call It Uranus?

Julie Sloane, "Mercury, Elements of the Ancients," accessed October 17, 2014, www.dartmouth
.edu/~toxmetal/mercury/history.html.

38. Kill Your Television . . . Except If Watching *Modern Family*

"Is Watching Too Much TV Making You Depressed?," accessed November 6, 2014, www
.elementsbehavioralhealth.com/featured/is-watching-too-much-tv-making-you-depressed.

39. Holy Mackerel!

"Indian Believers Swallow Live Fish as Asthma Cure," accessed September 5, 2014, www
.cbsnews.com/pictures/indian-believers-swallow-live-fish-as-asthma-cure.

40. Take the Lead. It's Prescription.

Jack Lewis, "Lead Poisoning: A Historical Perspective," accessed December 13, 2014, www2
.epa.gov/aboutepa/lead-poisoning-historical-perspective.

41. You Won't Always Be Able to Control Everything

"Choosing Baby Gender: Science versus Home Kits," accessed September 2, 2014, abcnews.go
.com/Technology/story?id=97287.

Owen D. Jones, "Sex Selection: Regulating Technology Enabling the Predetermination of a
Child's Gender," accessed August 23, 2014, jolt.law.harvard.edu/articles/pdf/v06
/06HarvJLTech001.pdf.

Suzanne Leigh, "Choosing Your Baby's Sex: What the Scientists Say," accessed August 28, 2014,
www.babycenter.com/0_choosing-your-babys-sex-what-the-scientists-say_2915.bc.

42. What If They Were Lactating?

Geoffrey Miller, Joshua M. Tybur, and Brent D. Jordan, "Ovulatory Effects on Tip Earnings by
Lap Dancers: Economic Evidence for Human Estrus?," accessed November 30, 2014, www
.unm.edu/~gfmiller/cycle_effects_on_tips.pdf.

43. Well, Who Is Going to Open the Pickle Jar?

"Coming Soon: Making Babies . . . without Sperm?," accessed January 7, 2015, theweek.com
/article/index/235881/coming-soon-making-babies-without-sperm.

Myranda Mowafi, "How Women Could Make Babies Without Men," accessed January 4,
2015, www.dailymail.co.uk/news/article-59196/How-women-make-babies-men.html.

44. Don't Blame the Irish

"Guinness Could Really Be Good for You?," accessed November 7, 2014, news.bbc.co.uk/2/hi
/3266819.stm.

"Why Did Doctors Prescribe Guinness to Pregnant Women?," accessed November 12, 2014,
gurumagazine.org/science/guinness-iron-pregnancy.

45. *And* It Makes You Look Cool

Janine K. Cataldo, Judith J. Prochaska, and Stanton A. Glantz, "Cigarette Smoking
Is a Risk Factor for Alzheimer's Disease: An Analysis Controlling for Tobacco
Industry Affiliation," *Journal of Alzheimer's Disease* 19, no. 2 (2010); doi:10.3233
/JAD-2010-1240.

"Smoking Prevents Alzheimer's? It Depends Who You Ask," accessed December 1, 2014, www
.theguardian.com/science/2010/mar/05/smoking-alzheimers-goldacre-bad-science.

46. Not Just Good for Serving Revenge

"Duct Tape More Effective than Cryotherapy for Warts," accessed October 29, 2014, www
.aafp.org/afp/2003/0201/p614.html.

Anjana Gosai, "Cold Comfort: Could You Cure Fatigue, Cellulite and Insomnia with Just Three Minutes in the Deep Freeze?," accessed October 27, 2014, www.dailymail.co.uk/femail /beauty/article-1329651/Cryotherapy-Could-cure-fatigue-cellulite-insomnia-just-minutes -deep-freeze.html#ixzz3J7raT4cW.

47. Does the Carpet Match the Drapes?

Michelle Healy, "Can Enzyme Supplements Really Keep Hair From Going Gray?," accessed January 4, 2015, www.usatoday.com/story/news/nation/2013/10/06/gray-hair-pills /2388619/.

"How to Prevent Gray Hair," accessed January 8, 2015, www.wikihow.com/Prevent-Gray -Hair.

"Powerful Grey Hair Natural Remedies," accessed January 5, 2015, www.life-saving -naturalcures-and-naturalremedies.com/grey-hair-natural-remedies.html.

48. We Are Not Suggesting You Suck on It

Sandy Calhoun Rice, "Breast Milk Protein Called Hamlet Helps Kill Dangerous Superbugs," accessed September 24, 2014, www.healthline.com/health-news/children-breast-milk -protein-kills-superbugs-050213.

"Substance in Breast Milk Kills Cancer Cells, Study Suggests," accessed September 23, 2014, www.sciencedaily.com/releases/2010/04/100419132403.htm.

"Substance Found in Breast Milk Kills 40 Types of Cancer Cells," accessed September 26, 2014, www.foxnews.com/story/2010/04/20/substance-found-in-breast-milk-kills-40-types-cancer -cells/.

50. Good for the Birds, Bad for the Worms

Jeff Grabmeier, "Procrastinators Get Poorer Grades in College Class, Study Finds," accessed October 14, 2014, researchnews.osu.edu/archive/procrast.htm.

Natalie Kitroeff, "Procrastination Is Bad for Your Grades," accessed October 13, 2014, www .businessweek.com/articles/2014-09-10/procrastination-is-bad-for-your-grades.

51. You Mean It Won't Fall Off?

Laura Berman, "The Health Benefits of Masturbation for Women and Men," accessed January 23, 2015, www.everydayhealth.com/sexual-health/dr-laura-berman-the-health -benefits-of-masturbation-for-women-and-men.aspx.

Maridel Reyes, "5 Reasons You Should Masturbate Tonight," accessed daily, www.menshealth .com/sex-women/masturbate-every-day.

52. How Many Licks Does It Take?

"The Sweat Test," accessed November 14, 2014, www.cff.org/aboutcf/testing/sweattest.

R. Busch, "On the History of Cystic Fibrosis," accessed November 15, 2014, www.ncbi.nlm .nih.gov/pubmed/2130674.

53. Try Not to Bruise It

Rebecca Wallersteiner, "Health Benefits of Reflexology," accessed December 1, 2014, www
.netdoctor.co.uk/healthy-living/complementary-health/health-benefits-of-reflexology.htm.

55. It's All in Your Head

Steven Novella, "Phrenology, History of a Pseudoscience," accessed January 5, 2015, www
.theness.com/index.php/phrenology-history-of-a-pseudoscience.

John van Wyhe, "The History of Phrenology," accessed January 3, 2015, www.victorianweb
.org/science/phrenology/intro.html.

56. Forget the Eye of the Tiger

Joseph Lin, "Top 10 Unusual Medical Treatments: Tiger Phallus Soup," accessed January 18,
2015, content.time.com/time/specials/packages/article/0,28804,1984400_1984439
_1984416,00.html.

Vanessa Woods, "Serving Up Hot Tiger Phallus Soup," accessed January 20, 2015,
dailyprincetonian.com/news/2002/04/serving-up-hot-tiger-phallus-soup.

57. They Eventually Get Their Revenge

www.businessinsider.com/warren-buffett-on-resume-building-2015-11. Accessed October 3, 2014.

Bonnie Malkin, "Male Science Nerds Most Likely to Be Virgins, Study Says," accessed October
7, 2014, www.telegraph.co.uk/news/worldnews/australiaandthepacific/australia/3547661
/Male-science-nerds-most-likely-to-be-virgins-study-says.html.

58. You Don't Need to Re-prove Gravity

L. Vanderford and M. Meyers, "Injuries and Bungee Jumping," accessed October 11, 2014,
www.ncbi.nlm.nih.gov/pubmed/8614758.

59. Are They Crooked?

"Chiropractic: An Introduction," accessed October 16, 2014, nccam.nih.gov/health
/chiropractic/introduction.htm.

"Chiropractic Care for Back Pain," accessed October 18, 2014, www.webmd.com/pain
-management/guide/chiropractic-pain-relief.

60. Dying for Sleep

"Study Ties 6–7 Hours of Sleep to Longer Life," accessed February 18, 2014, www.nytimes
.com/2002/02/15/us/study-ties-6-7-hours-of-sleep-to-longer-life.html.

61. Drinking to Improve Thinking

Annie Britton, Archana Singh-Manoux, and Michael Marmot, "Alcohol Consumption and
Cognitive Function in the Whitehall II Study," accessed February 21, 2014, aje
.oxfordjournals.org/content/160/3/240.full.

REFERENCES

62. Your Mane or Your Manliness?

Jennie Cohen, "9 Bizarre Baldness Cures," accessed August 23, 2014, www.history.com/news
/history-lists/9-bizarre-baldness-cures.

Wendy Demark-Wahnefried et al., "Early Onset Baldness and Prostate Cancer Risk," *Cancer
Epidemiology, Biomarkers & Prevention* 9 (2000): 325–28, cebp.aacrjournals.org
/content/913/325.full accessed August 23, 2014.

Lewis Lapham, ed., *Lapham's Quarterly* 2, no. 4 (Fall 2009), 170.

E. H. Ruddcok, MD, ed., *Vitalogy: An Encyclopedia of Health and Home* (Chicago: Vitalogy
Association, 1927), 82–85.

63. Paging Dr. Dracula

Gerry Greenstone, "The History of Bloodletting," *British Columbia Medical Journal* 52 (2010):
12–14.

Khosrow S. Houschyar et al., "Effects of Phlebotomy-Induced Reduction of Body Iron Stores
on Metabolic Syndrome: Results from a Randomized Clinical Trial," *BioMed Central
Medicine* 10 (2012): 54, accessed August 24, 2014, doi:10.1186/1741-7015-10-54.

"21st century bloodletting reduces cardiovascular risk," www.sciencedaily.com/releases
/2012/05/120529211645.htm. Accessed August 24, 2014.

Gilbert R. Seigworth, "Bloodletting over the Centuries," *New York State Journal of Medicine*
(1980): 2022–28.

64. Hurling at High Speed

Nicholas J. Wade, "The Original Spin Doctors—the Meeting of Perception and Insanity,"
Perception 34 (2005): 253–60.

65. Possibly a Posset for Parity?

Katrine Albertsen et al., "Alcohol Consumption during Pregnancy and the Risk of Preterm
Delivery," *American Journal of Epidemiology* 159 (2004): 155–61, accessed April 30,
2015, doi:10.1093/aje/kwh034.

J. L. Cook et al., "Progesterone and Prostaglandin H Synthase-2 Involvement in Alcohol-Induced
Preterm Birth in Mice," *Alcoholism Clinical and Experimental Research* 23 (1999): 1793–800.

Andy McDonald, "12 Disgusting Alcoholic Drinks We Dare You to Try. Triple Dog Dare You,"
accessed April 30, 2015, www.huffingtonpost.com/2013/10/10/gross-alcoholic-drinks_n
_4059712.html.

Meredith Franco Meyers, "Should You Drink Alcohol to Induce Labor?," accessed April 30,
2015, www.parents.com/pregnancy/my-body/is-it-safe/alcohol-induce-labor.

66. Parsley, Sage, Rosemary, and Thyme

"Apiol: Abortive and Toxic Effects," accessed November 2, 2015, flipper.diff.org/apprulesitems
/items/4756.

Kate Hermann, Anne Le Roux, and F. S. Fiddes, "Death from Apiol Used as Abortifacient,"
Lancet 270 (1956): 937–39.

Edward Shorter, *Women's Bodies: A Social History of Women's Encounter with Health, Ill-Health, and Medicine* (New Brunswick, NJ: Transaction Publishers, 1991), 213–24.

67. Finally, a Medical Reason to *Not* Exercise

Rachele Cooper, "How Can You Overdose on BenGay?," accessed May 4, 2015, scienceline.org /2007/08/ask-cooper-bengaydeath.

Gueorgi Kossinets and Duncan J. Watts, "Origins of Homophily in an Evolving Social Network," *American Journal of Sociology* 115 (2009): 411, accessed February 28, 2010, doi:10.1086/599247.

"Sports Cream Warnings Urged after Teen's Death," accessed May 4, 2015, www.nbcnews .com/id/19208195/ns/health-fitness/t/sports-cream-warnings-urged-after-teens-death/# .VUf2CWZla0c.

"Teen Dies from Muscle Cream Overdose," accessed May 4, 2015, www.foxnews.com/story /2007/06/09/teen-dies-from-muscle-cream-overdose.

68. Poor Pooh Bear

Grace Chua, "Bear Bile Still Prized as Traditional Remedy," accessed May 19, 2015, www .healthxchange.com.sg/News/Pages/Bear-bile-still-prized-as-traditional-remedy.aspx.

Andrew Jacobs, "Folk Remedy Extracted from Captive Bears Stirs Furor in China," accessed May 19, 2015, www.nytimes.com/2013/05/22/world/asia/chinese-bear-bile-farming-draws -charges-of-cruelty.html?pagewanted=all&_r=0.

Ben Kavoussi, "Asian Bear Bile Remedies: Traditional Medicine or Barbarism?," accessed May 19, 2015, www.sciencebasedmedicine.org/asian-bear-bile-remedies-barbarism-or -medicine.

69. And It Burns, Burns, Burns, the Ring of Fire . . .

Nader N. Massarweh, Ned Cosgriff, and Douglas P. Slakey, "Electrosurgery: History, Principles, and Current and Future Uses," *Journal of American College of Surgeons* 202 (2006): 520–30, accessed May 11, 2015, doi:10.1016.

Charles Donald O'Malley, *Andreas Vesalius of Brussels, 1514–1564* (California: University of California Press, 1964).

P. W. Soballe et al., "Electric Cautery Lowers the Contamination Threshold for Infection of Laparotomies," *American Journal of Surgery* 175 (1998): 263–66, accessed May 11, 2015. www.ncbinlm.nih.gov/pubmed/9568648.

Holly Tucker, "Early Surgery & Cautery: Or How to Boil a Puppy," accessed May 11, 2015, www.wondersandmarvels.com/2009/02/early-surgery-cautery-or-how-to-boil.html.

70. Snow in Your Nose

Miles Berry, *Allen Ginsberg: A Biography* (New York: Virgin Books, 2001).

Caleb Hellerman, "Cocaine: The Evolution of the Once 'Wonder' Drug," accessed April 23, 2015, www.cnn.com/2011/HEALTH/07/22/social.history.cocaine.

"Cocaine: A Brief History of Blow," accessed April 23, 2015, www.cbsnews.com/pictures
/cocaine-a-brief-history-of-blow/8.

"Position Statement: Medical Use of Cocaine," accessed April 23, 2015, www.entnet.org
/content/medical-use-cocaine.

71. Aspire to Respire, but Avoid to Not Expire

"Cigares de Joy," accessed May 16, 2015, thequackdoctor.com/index.php/cigares-de-joy.

"Epidemiologic Notes and Reports Jimson Weed Poisoning—Texas, New York, and California,
1994," accessed May 16, 2015, www.cdc.gov/mmwr/preview/mmwrhtml/00035694.htm.

E. Pretorius and J. Marx, "*Datura stramonium* in Asthma Treatment and Possible Effects on
Prenatal Development," *Environmental Toxicology and Pharmacology* 21, no. 3 (2006):
331–37, accessed May 16, 2015, doi:10.1016/j.etap.2005.10.006.

72. Liquidating Lousy Lice

Naomi Baumslag M.D. M.P.H.: *Nazi Doctors, Human Experimentation, and Typhus*. Praeger, 2005.

"DDT," accessed May 6, 2015, www.discoveriesinmedicine.com/Com-En/DDT.html.

"The US Army Used DDT to De-louse Soldiers," accessed November 2, 2015, www
.appalachianhistory.net/2015/07/army-used-ddt-for-de-lousing.html.

73. A Cup Should Not Go Up

Suzy Cohen, "Coffee Enema Benefits for You," accessed May 10, 2015, suzycohen.com
/?s=coffee+enema&submit.x=0&submit.y=0.

John W. Eisele and Donald T. Reay, "Deaths Related to Coffee Enemas," *Journal of the
American Medical Association* 244 (1980): 1608–9, accessed May 10, 2015,
doi:10.1001/jama.1980.03310140066036.

Scott Gavura, "Ask the (Science-Based) Pharmacist: What Are the Benefits of Coffee
Enemas?," accessed May 10, 2015, www.sciencebasedmedicine.org/ask-the-science-based
-pharmacist-what-are-the-benefits-of-coffee-enemas.

74. Lettin' Go Lentigo

"Home Remedies to Get Rid of Freckles," accessed April 28, 2015, www.top10homeremedies
.com/home-remedies/home-remedies-to-get-rid-of-freckles.html/3.

"Say Goodbye to Freckles With 9 Home Remedies," accessed April 28, 2015, www
.findhomeremedy.com/say-goodbye-to-freckles-with-9-home-remedies.

B. N. Sinha "Natural Ayurvedic Home Remedies for Freckles," accessed April 28, 2015, www
.homeveda.com/skin/natural-ayurvedic-home-remedies-for-freckles.html.

Yim Yiu-kin, "Being Freckle-Free," accessed April 28, 2015, www.joyousliving.hkhs.com/en
/joyous/wellness/119-2011-03-18-08-25-18.

75. Hashing Out Headbanging Hazards

Declan Patton and Andrew McIntosh, "Head and Neck Injury Risks in Heavy Metal: Head
Bangers Stuck between Rock and a Hard Bass," *BMJ* 337 (2008): 1–4, accessed May 13,
2015, doi:10.1136/bmj.a2825.

Ariyan Pirayesh Islamian, Manolis Polemikos, and Joachim K. Krauss, "Chronic Subdural Haematoma Secondary to Headbanging," *Lancet* 384 (2014): 102, accessed May 13, 2015, doi:10.1016/S0140-6736(14)60923-5.

Jordan Lite, "Head-Bangers, Beware of Injury, Rocker Scientists Warn," accessed May 13, 2015, blogs.scientificamerican.com/news-blog/head-bangers-beware-of-injury-rocke-2008-12-17.

76. Heroin: The All-Time Addictive, Snorting, Injecting, Smoking, Disorienting, Constipating, So-You-Can-Throw-It-All-Away Medicine

"DrugFacts: Heroin," accessed May 19, 2015, www.drugabuse.gov/publications/drugfacts/heroin.

Daven Hiskey, "The Pharmaceutical Company Bayer Coined the Name 'Heroin' and Marketed the Drug as a Non-Addictive Cough Medicine," accessed May 19, 2015, www.todayifoundout.com/index.php/2012/02/the-pharmaceutical-company-bayer-coined-the-name-heroin-and-marketed-the-drug-as-a-non-addictive-cough-medicine.

"Yes, Bayer Promoted Heroin for Children—Here Are the Ads That Prove It," accessed May 19, 2015, www.businessinsider.com/yes-bayer-promoted-heroin-for-children-here-are-the-ads-that-prove-it-2011-11.

77. Halting Harassing Hiccups

"Calvin and Hobbes," accessed May 13, 2015, www.gocomics.com/calvinandhobbes/2010/06/02.

Full-Young Chang and Ching-Liang Lu, "Hiccup: Mystery, Nature and Treatment," *Journal of Neurogastroenterology and Motility* 18 (2012): 123–30, accessed May 13, 2015, doi:10.5056/jnm.2012.18.2.123.

Lewis H. Lapham, ed., *Lapham's Quarterly* 11 (2009): 139.

"Longest Attack of Hiccups," accessed May 13, 2015, news.bbc.co.uk/2/shared/spl/hi/pop_ups/05/health_guinness_medical_record_breakers/html/2.stm.

78. The Importance of Impotence

Chris Iliades, "11 Wackiest Erectile Dysfunction 'Cures' of All Time," accessed May 11, 2015, www.everydayhealth.com/erectile-dysfunction-pictures/wackiest-erectile-dysfunction-cures-of-all-time.aspx#07.

Angus McLaren, *Impotence: A Cultural History*. University of Chicago Press, 2007.

Angus McLaren, "Two Millennia of Impotence Cures," accessed May 11, 2015, www.press.uchicago.edu/Misc/Chicago/500768.html.

79. When the Treatment Is Worse Than the Disease

Insulin Coma Therapy: www.pbs.org/wgbh/amex/nosh/filmore/ps_ict.html.

David Hay Jones, "Insulin Coma Therapy," accessed May 4, 2015, www.typ1diabetes.com/insulin_shock_therapy.htm.

Dora Kohen, "Diabetes Mellitus and Schizophrenia: Historical Perspective," *British Journal of Psychiatry* 184 (2004): s64–s66, accessed May 4, 2015, doi:10.1192/bjp.184.47.s64.

"Primary Sources: Insulin Coma Therapy," accessed May 4, 2015, www.pbs.org/wgbh/amex /nash/filmmore/ps_ict.html.

80. I'd Rather Have a Bottle in Front of Me Than a Frontal Lobotomy

"Moniz Develops Lobotomy for Mental Illness 1935," accessed May 9, 2015, www.pbs.org /wgbh/aso/databank/entries/dh35lo.html.

Tanya Lewis, "Lobotomy: Definition, Procedure and History," accessed May 9, 2015, www .livescience.com/42199-lobotomy-definition.html.

Tony Long, "Nov. 12, 1935: You Should (Not) Have a Lobotomy," accessed May 9, 2015, www.wired.com/2010/11/1112first-lobotomy.

81. To Do or Not

E. H. Ruddcok, ed., *Vitalogy: An Encyclopedia of Health and Home* (Chicago: Vitalogy Assocication, 1927), 898–99.

82. Take Two Skulls and Call Me in the Morning

Philip Bethge, "Europe's 'Medicinal Cannibalism': The Healing Power of Death," accessed May 5, 2015, www.spiegel.de/international/zeitgeist/europe-s-medicinal-cannibalism-the -healing-power-of-death-a-604548.html.

"Mirror, Mirror on the Wall, 2014 Update: How the U.S. Health Care System Compares Internationally," accessed May 5, 2015, www.commonwealthfund.org/publications/fund -reports/2014/jun/mirror-mirror.

Keith Veronese, "The Uncomfortably Common Practice of Medicinal Cannibalism," accessed May 5, 2015, io9.com/5971342/the-uncomfortably-common-practice-of-medicinal-cannibalism.

83. Itching to Add Inches

"Noninvasive Extenders Are Better Than Surgery for Men Who Want a Longer Penis, Study Finds," accessed May 19, 2015, www.sciencedaily.com/releases/2011/04/110418093842.htm.

"Penis-Enlargement Products: Do They Work?," accessed May 19, 2015, www.mayoclinic.org /healthy-lifestyle/sexual-health/in-depth/penis/art-20045363?pg=1.

David Veale et al., "Am I Normal? A Systematic Review and Construction of Nomograms for Flaccid and Erect Penis Length and Circumference in Up to 15,521 Men," *British Journal of Urology International* 115 (2015): 978–86, accessed May 19, 2015, doi:10.1111/bju.13010.

84. Pacifying Mr. Gandhi and Quieting Mister Ed

"Five-Year Findings of the Hypertension Detection and Follow-Up Program. I. Reduction in Mortality of Persons with High Blood Pressure, Including Mild Hypertension. Hypertension Detection and Follow-Up Program Cooperative Group," *Journal of the American Medical Association.* 242 (1979): 2562–71.

"Herbs that Help Lower High Blood Pressure / Hypertension," accessed May 4, 2015, www
.medindia.net/patients/lifestyleandwellness/herbs-for-high-blood-pressure-indian-snakeroot
.htm.

"Medicine: Pills for Mental Illness?," accessed May 4, 2015, content.time.com/time/magazine
/article/0,9171,857672,00.html.

Reserpine use on horses: egnimed.com/drugs-and-medications/reference/reserpine. Accessed
December 19, 2014.

85. Everybody Gettin' Horny

Peter Gwin, "Rhino Wars," *National Geographic,* March 2012.

"Rhino Horn Use: Fact vs. Fiction," accessed April 30, 2015, www.pbs.org/wnet/nature
/rhinoceros-rhino-horn-use-fact-vs-fiction/1178/.

86. Click It or Ticket!

David Bjerklie, "The Hidden Danger of Seat Belts," accessed May 4, 2015, content.time.com
/time/nation/article/0,8599,1564465,00.html.

Alma Cohen and Liran Einav, "The Effects of Mandatory Seat Belt Laws on Driving Behavior
and Traffic Fatalities," *Review of Economics and Statistics* 85 (2003): 828–43.

"Did You Know?," accessed May 4, 2015, www.ama-assn.org/ama/pub/about-ama/our-history
/did-you-know.page?.

"Seat Belts: Get the Facts," accessed May 4, 2015, www.cdc.gov/motorvehiclesafety/seatbelts
/facts.html.

Malcolm J. Wardlaw, "Three Lessons for a Better Cycling Future," *BMJ* 321 (2000): 1582–85.

87. Sleep Divorce to Prevent Real Divorce?

"More Couples Opting to Sleep in Separate Beds, Study Suggests," accessed May 6, 2015, www
.cbc.ca/news/health/more-couples-opting-to-sleep-in-separate-beds-study-suggests-1.1316019.

Andrea Petersen, "Who Sleeps Better at Night?," *Wall Street Journal,* June 4, 2012, accessed
May 6, 2015, www.wsj.com/news/articles/SB100014240527023038302045774463425155
28860.

"Separate Beds Are Liberating," accessed May 6, 2015, www.salon.com/2012/08/14/separate
_beds_are_liberating/?utm_source=huffpost_women&utm_medium=referral&utm_
campaign=pubexchange_article.

88. Doctor's Orders: Twelve Bottles of Beer, by Mouth, Daily

"Library Treasures: Dover on Sydenham's Smallpox Treatment," accessed May 9, 2015, www
.historyofvaccines.org/content/blog/library-treasures-dover-sydenhams-smallpox-treatment.

Albert S. Lyons and R. Joseph Petrucelli II, *Medicine—An Illustrated History* (New York:
Abradale Press, Harry N. Abrams Inc., 1987).

James C. Moore, *The History of the Smallpox* (London: Longman, 1815).

REFERENCES

Stefan Riedel, "Edward Jenner and the History of Smallpox and Vaccination," *Proceedings of Baylor University Medical Center* 18 (2005): 21–25.

89. Beating the Stick

"Health Effects of Cigarette Smoking," accessed on May 19, 2015, www.cdc.gov/tobacco/data _statistics/fact_sheets/health_effects/effects_cig_smoking/index.htm.

Douglas E. Jorenby et al., "A Controlled Trial of Sustained-Release Bupropion, a Nicotine Patch, or Both for Smoking Cessation," *New England Journal of Medicine* 340 (1999): 685–91, accessed May 19, 2015.

Emily Kaufman, "Quitter Jitters? 14 Natural Ways to Stop Smoking," accessed May 19, 2015, www.today.com/health/natural-ways-stop-smoking-1D80227639.

90. No Wrinkle in Chyme?

"Gastric Cancer Treatment—for Health Professionals," accessed April 24, 2015, www.cancer .gov/cancertopics/pdq/treatment/gastric/HealthProfessional.

Lizzie Parry, "Botox Could Be Used as New Treatment for Stomach Cancer as Scientists Discover Anti-wrinkle Treatment Slows Tumour Growth," *Daily Mail*, August 20, 2014, accessed April 24, 2015, www.dailymail.co.uk/health/artcile-2729972/Botox-used-new -treatment-stomach-cancer-experts-say-html.

E. H. Ruddock, ed., *Vitalogy: An Encyclopedia of Health and Home.* Chicago: Vitalogy Association, 1922.

Chun-Mei Zhao et al., "Denervation Suppresses Gastric Tumorigenesis," *Science Translational Medicine* 6 (2014), accessed April 24, 2015, doi:10.1126/scitranslmed.3009569.

91. Honey, I Healed the Wound!

A. B. Jull, N. Walker, and S. Deshpande. "Honey as a Topical Treatment for Wounds," Cochrane Database Systematic Reviews, accessed August 14, 2014, www.ncbi.nlm.nih.gov/pubmed /23450557.

Katherine Harmon, "Honey Helps Health Wounds," accessed August 17, 2014, www .scientificamerican.com/podcast/episode/honey-helps-heal-wounds-12-01-31.

92. The Sad Story and Salvation of Thalidomide

Bara Fintel, Athena T. Samaras, and Edson Carias, "The Thalidomide Tragedy: Lessons for Drug Safety and Regulation," accessed May 4, 2015, helix.northwestern.edu/article /thalidomide-tragedy-lessons-drug-safety-and-regulation.

Ananya Mandal, "History of Thalidomide," accessed May 4, 2015, www.news-medical.net /health/History-of-Thalidomide.aspx.

Michael Winerip, "The Death and Afterlife of Thalidomide," *New York Times,* September 23, 2013, accessed May 4, 2015, www.nytimes.com/2013/09/23/booming/the-death-and -afterlife-of-thalidomide.html?_r=0.

93. Finding *Frankenstein*'s Fountainhead

Miss Celania, "Who Was Dr. Frankenstein?," accessed May 6, 2015, mentalfloss.com/article
   /19855/who-was-dr-frankenstein.

Jennifer Latson, "Did a Real-Life Alchemist Inspire *Frankenstein*?," accessed May 6, 2015,
   time.com/3648440/mary-shelley-frankenstein-history.

Roseanne Montillo, "The Gruesome, True Inspiration Behind 'Frankenstein,'" accessed May 6,
   2015, www.huffingtonpost.com/roseanne-montillo/the-gruesome-true-inspira_b_2622633
   .html.

94. Guess I'll Go Eat Worms

Ferris Jabr, "For the Good of the Gut: Can Parasitic Worms Treat Autoimmune Diseases?,"
   accessed February 18, 2015, www.scientificamerican.com/article/helminthic-therapy-mucus.

Rachel Nuwer, "Worm Therapy: Why Parasites May Be Good for You," accessed February 18,
   2015, www.bbc.com/future/story/20130422-feeling-ill-swallow-a-parasite.

95. One of the Few Practices We Endorse

"Get Bigger Breasts without Surgery," accessed September 30, 2014, www.wikihow.com/Get
   -Bigger-Breasts-Without-Surgery.

Jordin Keim, "Ways to Make Your Breasts Grow," accessed October 2, 2014, beauty
   .allwomenstalk.com/ways-to-make-your-breasts-grow.

96. Getting Pissy

Bret Easton Ellis, *American Psycho*. New York: Vintage Books, 1991.

Jill McGivering, "Thais Drink Urine as Alternative Medicine," accessed June 21, 2015, news
   .bbc.co.uk/2/hi/asia-pacific/3083577.stm.

Index